Professional Care

Alastair V. Campbell

PROFESSIONAL CARE

Its Meaning and Practice

FORTRESS PRESS Philadelphia

First published in 1984 by SPCK, London, England, and
Fortress Press, Philadelphia, Pennsylvania, U.S.A.

Library of Congress Cataloging in Publication Data
Campbell, Alastair V.
   Professional care.
   Bibliography: p.
   Includes index.
   1. Medicine—Religious aspects—Christianity—
Addresses, essays, lectures. 2. Social service—
Religious aspects—Christianity—Addresses, essays,
lectures. I. Title.
BT732.C28 1984   261.5′6   84-4081
ISBN 0-8006-1812-2

K898A84   Printed in the United Kingdom   1-1812

Contents

Acknowledgements   vi

Preface   vii

Preamble   1

1. Lovers and Professors   5

2. Medical Power   17

3. Nursing, Nurturing and Sexism   34

4. The Two Faces of Social Work   52

5. The Claim to Purity   70

6. Knowing What is Best   87

7. Caring and Being Cared For   101

8. The Politics of Love   115

Notes   128

Select Bibliography   142

Index   145

Acknowledgements

The publishers acknowledge permission to quote from the following copyright sources:

W.H. Auden: excerpts from 'The Shield of Achilles', in *Collected Poems*. Reprinted by permission of Faber & Faber and Random House, Inc.

Charles Causley: an excerpt from 'Ten Types of Hospital Visitor', in *Collected Poems 1971-75*. Reprinted by permission of Macmillan.

T.S. Eliot: excerpts from 'Ash Wednesday' and 'Four Quartets', in *Collected Poems 1909-1962*. Reprinted by permission of Faber & Faber and Harcourt Brace Jovanovich, Inc.

R.D. Laing: an excerpt from *Knots*. Reprinted by permission of Tavistock Publications and Random House Inc. (Pantheon Books).

Paris Leary: excerpts from 'He's Frightfully Good at Coping', in *Views of the Oxford Colleges and Other Poems*. Copyright © 1960 by Paris Leary. Reprinted by permission of Charles Scribner's Sons.

Louis MacNeice: an excerpt from 'Prayer Before Birth', in *The Collected Poems of Louis MacNeice*. Reprinted by permission of Faber & Faber.

Edwin Muir: excerpts from 'One Foot in Eden' and 'The Transfiguration', in *The Collected Poems of Edwin Muir*. Copyright © 1960 by Willa Muir. Reprinted by permission of Faber & Faber and Oxford University Press, Inc.

Anne Sexton: an excerpt from 'Doctors', in *An Awful Rowing Towards God*. Copyright © 1975 by Loring Conant, Jr. Reprinted by permission of Houghton Mifflin Company and The Sterling Lord Agency, Inc.

Rabindranath Tagore: an excerpt from 'The Gardener'. Reprinted by permission of Macmillan.

Leo Tolstoy: excerpts from 'The Death of Ivan Ilyich', in *The Cossacks and Other Stories*, translated by Rosemary Edmonds. Copyright © 1960 by Rosemary Edmonds. Reprinted by permission of Penguin Books Ltd.

Preface

This book contains the substance of the Edward Cadbury
Lectures which I delivered in the University of Birmingham in
the Spring Term of 1983. I have substantially revised and re-
ordered the lectures in preparation for publication and have
provided a detailed list of references to aid readers who wish to
pursue at greater depth any of the issues discussed.

The Edward Cadbury Lectureship was established in 1941
by Edward Cadbury Esquire, LL.D. for the furtherance of the
study of Theology in the University of Birmingham. According
to the regulations there shall be an annual course of Lectures,
usually eight in number, to be delivered in either the Autumn
or Spring Term. The theme of the Lectures shall be concerned
with some aspect of the Christian faith, the original intention
of the Founder being that it should be concerned with the
relations past, present and future, of Christianity to civilization
and culture. The theme I have selected is intended to honour
this intention by considering insights from Christian theology
into a notable phenomenon of contemporary life, the rise of
professionalism in caring.

It is customary in prefaces to acknowledge one's indebtedness
to others, but in the case of this book this acknowledgement is
demanded by more than mere politeness. I trespassed so far
into other people's academic territory in preparing the lectures
that I found myself frequently drawing on the resources of
others in order to find my bearings. I feel myself very fortunate
in being a member of a university in which research at a high
level is carried out in the professionally orientated disciplines
and in which disciplinary boundaries are so easily crossed. For
detailed help and advice I am especially grateful to Annie
Altschul, Stewart Asquith, Chris Clark and Lesley Hardy. I
have received additional stimulus from the work of two former
students of mine, Marilyn Ross and Stephen Pattison. I would

Preface

also like to express my thanks to the many colleagues in Birmingham University who offered hospitality, encouragement and positive criticism, in particular Gordon and Mary Davies and Michael and Jean Wilson.

During the period of the lectures and the revision for publication I received outstanding secretarial help from Alison Johnson and (most especially) Elma Webster, who tolerated my changes of phrase beyond any reasonable expectation. This final outcome of much labour and much goodwill from friends and colleagues is dedicated to Elma as a tribute to another kind of (often unrecognized) professionalism.

Edinburgh, July 1983.

Preamble

This book consists of an exploration in eight parts of the theological dimensions of the professional care offered by doctors, nurses and social workers. Since this is a somewhat unusual project it may be subject to some misunderstandings, which should be cleared up before the beginning of the exploration.

First, my choice of the professions of medicine, nursing and social work may be regarded as somewhat arbitrary and insecurely founded in a theory of professionalism. The very term 'profession' is the subject of a complex and continuing debate within sociological theory,[1] and of the three 'professions' I have selected only medicine would satisfy the criteria of some sociological definitions.[2] I have chosen, however, to disregard these debates and to see it as sufficient that these three occupational groups make *claims* to be professions, claims which are widely accepted by the lay public who grant them employment and statutory recognition. My selection of these three specific groups has been determined by their close involvement with health and welfare services and thereby with people who are in an especially vulnerable situation. Obviously there are many other groups who also claim to deal professionally with people when they are in a state of vulnerability or need. The list of such groups could be very extensive, including lawyers, school teachers, probation officers, housing officials, therapists of numerous kinds, police officers, funeral directors and ancillary health workers. My choice of doctors, nurses and social workers is certainly radically selective, but it has not been merely arbitrary. Two factors have determined my choice: (1) these three professions have produced extensive theoretical discussions of the nature of their professional practice; (2) these professions deal in a more wide-ranging manner with people in need than the other occupational

1

groups I have mentioned. (The boundaries of their professional authority and competence are not so clearly defined as those of, say, a policeman, a schoolteacher or a funeral director.)

Taking such factors into account, I might well have included another occupational group not so far mentioned in my list – the clergy. This is a group which deals with people professionally in times of vulnerability and need and within ill-defined boundaries. I have excluded them, however, because I believe they merit a separate study of a different type. The professional status of ministers is a more contentious one than that of 'secular' professions, because of theological considerations relating to 'vocation' and to the ministry of all believers. Thus the theological task of exploring their offering of care is a different one from that attempted in this volume.[3] I am left, therefore, with medicine, nursing and social work as the professions (or claimants to professional status) most central to my interest in the theology of professional care.

A second potential misunderstanding relates to the explicitly religious orientation of this study. It might appear that I am writing exclusively for those who share the Christian beliefs which have shaped my explorations. This is most certainly not my intention. I am not directing my observations only to Christian social workers, nurses and doctors. Rather I am offering theological reflections on concerns which cross divisions between believers and non-believers. I do not expect every reader to agree with all my speculations, or indeed to make sense of all the religious imagery, some of which may be obscured by the inevitable use of 'in-group' language to describe it. But I must emphasize that lack of religious belief, or commitment to a religion other than Christianity, should not be seen as a barrier to reading this book and engaging in intellectual debate with its arguments. I have tried to write in a language which communicates with all who are willing to think speculatively or adventurously, for this, I am convinced, should be the aim of all theological writing, but most especially of my particular discipline, Practical Theology.

Thirdly, my colleagues in theology, especially perhaps those who specialize in Systematic Theology, may observe with some disquiet that (in the latter part of the book particularly) I expropriate and reinterpret major theological doctrines with a

2

minimum of scholarly justification. This somewhat cavalier approach (no doubt it is a mistake to offer one's critics such a telling phrase!) is one to which I readily confess. My use of theological ideas has been deliberately associative and possibly idiosyncratic, because I regard my task as one of creating imaginative links between religious and non-religious interpretations of professionalism. For this reason I have described this volume as '*A* Theology of Professional Care'. I speak of 'explorations' and not of 'explanations'. It may well be that I have missed some signs and that I stumble from time to time into quagmires of my own confusions. Nevertheless, I hope that my readers, whether theologically informed or not, will find that this essay in Practical Theology opens some interesting new vistas on the transcendent character of human caring.

ONE

Lovers and Professors

Suffer us not to mock ourselves with falsehood
Teach us to care and not to care
Teach us to sit still
     T.S. Eliot, *Ash Wednesday*[1]

1. LOVE OR SELF-ADVANCEMENT?

There is, at least, an ambiguity and, at worst, a deep dishonesty in the notion of professional care. Other people's ill-health, confusion and social disadvantage are sources of power, status and income for those groups in society who offer their services as professional helpers. What then are we to make of the high-sounding ethical codes of such self-styled 'caring professions'? Are they mocking themselves (or perhaps more likely their patients and clients) with falsehood? Helen Gardner has spoken of a delicate balance between indifference and detachment in Eliot's *Ash Wednesday*, from which my opening quotation comes.[2] But could such delicacy possibly be applied to paid, professional relationships? Or is this a false (perhaps a treacherous) idealism?

The ambiguous title of this chapter, with its hints of academic indiscretions,[3] is meant to dramatize this odd juxtaposition of service and personal advantage. I have chosen the title to disclose how strange it is that certain occupational groups *profess* to *love*, claiming both the title 'profession' and a commitment to 'service of mankind'. These groups are both 'lovers' and 'professors', it seems. Indeed, what they profess, in addition to knowledge and skill, *is* disinterested love. They are set apart from other occupational groups, including other professions, by being described as 'welfare professions', 'caring professions', 'helping professions', or, in a phrase coined by

5

Paul Halmos, 'personal service professions'.[4] They promise to deliver not just physical treatment or material aid, but (in another phrase of Halmos') a 'tenderness [which] absorbs manipulation'.[5] They profess to deal with people not simply by the rules of fair trading (as any seller of services should), but also by an ethic of 'respect for persons'.

Yet is the word 'love' really the right one in this context? After all, it is rarely, if ever, used by doctors, nurses or social workers themselves to describe their professional relationships with patients or clients. What they promise is a consistent, skilled and informed concern, including a respect for individual dignity and rights. Such professional commitments, it may be argued, are not to be confused with love, a personal relationship, which (as Kant claimed so forcibly)[6] cannot be commanded. Nevertheless, if love is fully understood in all its moral and theological complexity (an issue to which I shall be returning in some detail later), then consistent professional care *is* a form of love. It entails a personal commitment by the person offering care which cannot be captured solely in the language of contract. I shall be suggesting that, only if we view professional care as a form of 'moderated love', can we do justice to its special character.

Such an approach may appear psychologically and politically naive. Is there not a danger of being deceived by what is merely the rhetoric of professional self-advancement? In *Commitment to Welfare* Richard Titmuss observed that we might well regard professions as 'associations for spreading the gospel of self importance'.[7] It is a point which has been made many times over by writers in different fields. Bernard Shaw described professions as 'conspiracies against the laity';[8] Ivan Illich tirelessly accuses professionals of disabling their clients by accumulating inappropriate authority;[9] and Paul Wilding in *Professional Power and Social Welfare* describes professional codes of ethics as 'campaign documents prepared in a search for privilege and power'.[10] Why then should I regard the professions' statements of disinterested concern for humanity as genuinely moral commitments?

There can be no simple answer to this question. It is obvious that self-interest enters into professional work, as it does into any occupation. Apart from financial security and emotional satisfaction, there is the important benefit of professional status and privilege. Wilding has pointed out that occupational groups which successfully gain professional status within a society have four privileges safeguarded: a state-enforced monopoly of the task they carry out; control of entry to the profession, both in terms of selection of candidates and of fixing a limit to overall numbers; control of length and content of training for the task; and determination of conditions of work.[11] In order to obtain such privileges (which may be summed up in the phrase 'professional autonomy') Wilding suggests that professions offer guarantees of their trustworthiness and their commitment to the common good by the promulgation of an ethical code and by disciplining their delinquent members. Thus an ethic which promises to serve the good of mankind plainly serves the good of the profession, especially if the 'good of mankind' is interpreted in ways which offer no serious challenges to the distribution of wealth, power and status within the society which licenses the profession.

Wilding's analysis cannot be lightly dismissed, but we should notice that it gains much of its force from the assumption that an explanation in egoistic terms is sufficient in itself. I wish to avoid the kind of reductionist approach which gives no weight at all to altruistic motivation. I agree that we may reasonably assume that no human acts can be found to be wholly disinterested, whether in a professional context or in any other. But the point to be established about professional care is not whether there are egoistic elements within it, but whether it is *only* a self-seeking activity, or so predominately a self-seeking one that the claim to be concerned for others is mere sham. It may well turn out that professionalism has nothing to do with love, but we must not suppose this to be self-evidently so simply because there is a gain for practitioners in being regarded as ethical.

2. PROFESSIONAL CARE AS LOVE

The idea that certain forms of professional care can be seen as the offering of love has been most fully developed by the sociologist, Paul Halmos. His last three books, *The Faith of the Counsellors*, *The Personal Service Society*, and *The Personal and the Political*, were all concerned with an understanding of the nature of the relationship which certain professions offer to patients or clients. Halmos believed that the ethical commitment of these 'personal service professions' should be taken as genuine, but that it also had to be seen as paradoxical in character, an orientation closer to religious faith than to scientific detachment. I shall examine Halmos' views in some detail, since they provide the reference points for my own exploration of the theology of professional care.

In *The Faith of the Counsellors* Halmos intended to describe and analyse a social phenomenon which had become very evident in the 1960s. He called it 'the coming of the counsellors'. Halmos had in mind not any single profession, but a group of people drawn from a range of professions, in particular medicine, social work and clinical psychology, who believed in the method of 'talking cures'.[12] Halmos considered that this group had a common ancestor in the clergyman, and a common aim for 'health, sanity, a state of unspecified virtue, even a state of grace, or merely a return to the virtues of the community'.[13] He saw this group as the successors to the diminishing number of priests, clergy and Religious in modern society, sharing as they did 'an unconfessed hope' in 'a kind of humanistic Kingdom of God'.[14]

The focus of attention in this book is on a full analysis of this unconfessed hope, which Halmos describes as the 'faith of the counsellors'. By means of an exhaustive survey of the literature of psychotherapy, social casework and counselling, he claims that counsellors act on the basis of several contradictory propositions, or antinomies. The one to which he gives most emphasis is the belief in love as therapeutic skill. The contradiction is obvious: counsellors argue for the use of a loving relationship in order to effect a cure, but how can love, a spontaneous emotional response, be regarded as a therapeutic technique? Halmos refuses to resolve this paradox, arguing that 'creative dissonance' is necessary in such helping professions, since they ultimately must depend not on science but on faith, and the essence of faith is paradox. The fact that the counsellors are most likely to deny this paradoxical element he takes as further proof that it exists![15]

In the last chapter of *The Faith of the Counsellors* Halmos begins to draw wider conclusions about the emergent counselling ideology, suggesting that it may be contributing towards a growth of love in society as a whole by encouraging the realization of humanistic values. These ideas are more fully developed in *The Personal Service Society*. In this book Halmos shifts his perspective somewhat and, instead of singling out a group of 'counsellors', he now identifies a number of professions as 'personal service professions'. (He places in this category clergy, doctors, nurses, teachers and social workers.) All these professions have, he believes, fallen under the moral influence of the counselling ideology described in his previous book. The personal service professions are to be distinguished from the impersonal service professions (e.g. lawyers, accountants, architects) by the fact that their 'principle function is to bring about changes in the body or personality of the client'.[16] Halmos thought that it was from such professions that the 'moral leadership' of post-industrial society would increasingly come. This was so because the personal service professional must learn to play a role which combines knowledge and skill with empathy and integrity. In such skilled altruism personal service professionals were providing a paradigm of love, which also served self-interest (the professionals' own career advancement). They could be seen as the new culture heroes upon whom people would learn to model their own moral ideals. Thus, although Halmos did not deny elements of self-interest inherent in the professional status, he remained confident that this did not contradict the role of the personal service professions as principal carriers of a moral idealism, which combined egoism and altruism.[17]

It will be clear even from these brief summaries that the tone of these two books is markedly optimistic. Halmos leaves one in little doubt that he himself shares the belief which he has identified as the foundation of the counsellors' creed – 'faith in the triumph of love over hatred'.[18] His last book, however, was very different in mood and style. Entitled *The Personal and the Political: Social Work and Political Action*, it revealed the author's awareness of the shift in emphasis in social work practice and theory from social casework (itself influenced by what has been called 'the psychoanalytic deluge')[19] towards community development and political action. Halmos appeared

9

to view this change with a mixture of trepidation and disgust, and much of his book was an attack on the 'spirit of recalcitrance' which he believed the radical social work theorists were promoting. Alarmed by attempts to find a synthesis of the personal and the political (and more especially by the 'politicization of the personal' of Marxist theorists) Halmos' new concern was to '*reassert* the moral respectability of caution'.[20] He repeated the idea of faith based on paradoxes, believing that only such a *coincidentia oppositorum* could moderate political extremism and 'cultivate poise and gentle balance'.[21]

A constant theme of this last book is the incompatibility of the personal and the political. Attempts to mix them will result in the loss of the essential features of one or the other, and most likely of the personal, because this is the 'softer' one. Each individual helper must be prepared to see the validity of both approaches, and, if his personality inclines him to follow one, he should at least try to learn from the other and to tolerate those for whom it is the more important. Halmos uses the image of the tightrope walker, who harnesses the forces of gravity on either side of him to allow him to maintain balance and move forward.[22] Thus he can find no place for the political within the faith of the counsellor. The political is seen as alien to love, a separate reality, a counterpoise to personal caring.

3. THE THEOLOGY OF LOVE

These analyses of professionalism by Halmos have received much praise and much criticism. They may be seen as virtually unique in the detailed attention devoted to the character of professional care and as prophetic in identifying evaluative or 'faith' elements in professionalism before such a perception became commonplace. Criticism has focused on his sociology of professionalization and on his attack on radical social work. The former is, to say the least, idiosyncratic, and seems to depend on rather loosely defined categories.[23] The latter can be seen as both incomplete and partisan.[24] It is his appeal to theology, however, which is of especial interest to my theme. He is unsparing in the use of terms like 'faith', 'belief',

10

'vocation'. In all three books he draws explicit parallels between Christian values and professional values. (For example, in *The Faith of the Counsellors* he writes: '. . . the works of counselling are more Christian than most practices of our times, even if the counsellor's puritanism forbids him the easy solace of naive and pious fantasies'.)[25] Yet from a theological perspective his discussion of faith, of Christian values, and most especially of love, is not adequate. By showing how Halmos' treatment of love is incomplete theologically, I shall be able to map out the issues with which the rest of this book will be concerned. There are weaknesses in Halmos' exposition of professional care as 'love' in the following four areas: (1) the meaning of 'love'; (2) love of self and love of others; (3) love and justice; and (4) the transcendent element in love.

(1) *The meaning of 'love'*

The most obvious weakness in Halmos' arguments is that, although 'love' is a key term for him (especially in *The Faith of the Counsellors*), he does not offer any proper definition, nor does he even pay adequate attention to the ambiguity of the term. No doubt this is partly the fault of the sources he is summarizing. Much counselling literature refers somewhat vaguely to 'love', 'warmth', 'positive regard', without acknowledging the complexities entailed. But, if Halmos wishes to identify a paradoxical relationship between spontaneous feelings and planned professional technique, it is essential that he clarify what is meant by 'love'. To some extent he may be offering an answer in terms of the professional's role-playing which is (or may become) authentic altruistic concern. Yet, again, the relationship between reason and emotion in such role-playing remains unclear.

My first task, therefore, must be to look in considerable detail at the caring relationship in the three professions I have selected for study (medicine, nursing and social work), in order to find ways of clarifying the character of the love imputed to them. This will occupy our attention in the next three chapters, and we shall find that it is by no means easy to disentangle the different elements involved. In particular, the need for rationality and detachment in professional work makes the notion of love in such relationships both elusive and ambiguous.

(2) *Love of self and love of others*

Implicit in the problem of speaking of professional work as love is the question of the relationship between self-interest and altruism. Halmos refers to this issue on a number of occasions, but fails to grasp the nettle of the seeming conflict between these two loves. For example, he writes (in *The Personal Service Society*) this somewhat perverse sentence:

> Of course, the professional role does not void the self and its inviolable compact with itself; it merely makes the self serve itself in an entirely novel way by making it act selfishly in an unselfish manner.[26]

To the extent that this statement represents a refusal to draw a radical contrast between egoism and altruism, it is helpful, but only minimally so. Halmos makes it plain that moral progress must come not by reducing selfishness but by transforming it. Implicit here is a notion of the 'true self' which finds its fulfilment by an escape from competitive self-seeking into a life of service. We must ask (much more radically than Halmos does) whether such a possibility is a real one in society as we know it. As I have already observed, a convincing case can be made out for the view that the seeming altruism of professionals is a luxury they can readily afford, when there is no real challenge to their social status, professional privilege and material security in acting in this manner. Disinterested concern is manifest only when there is a real cost to the self in expressing it. Thus what I shall describe as 'the claim to purity' of the professions needs exploring within the context of a full theoretical discussion of the relationships between self-interest, sympathy and altruism. This task will be undertaken in chapter 5.

(3) *Love and justice*

We are led naturally from the problem of self-interest to the question of the relationship between love and justice. The polemical tone of Halmos' last book seems to betray a failure to see the importance of this issue. By polarizing the 'social reformers' and the 'personal carers' Halmos makes it impossible to consider the possibility that love may express itself in social justice, not only in one-to-one encounters. He is of course aware of attempts to make such a synthesis, using as examples some of the Latin American liberation theologians,[27] but, because he has failed to discuss the meaning of 'love' adequately, he cannot understand what is being attempted by such theorists. Had Halmos begun with an exploration of the concept of neighbour-love (*agape*) as equal regard for all human beings, he might have come to the realization that political involvement and love-as-*agape* are inseparable. His approach seems to trap professionals into insulating their socio-political awareness from their professional life, while failing to realize that all socially significant action is inevitably political in character. Only if professional work had no social effect at all could it be regarded as exempt from political issues.

Any attempt to correct Halmos' bias is itself subject to difficulty, because his perception that professional care and political awareness are uneasy bedfellows is certainly correct. Many contemporary theologians see love and justice as inseparable, but experience great problems in describing the practical implications of this view for an ethic based on respect for each individual. We shall see the problem highlighted in social work theory (chapter 4) and will return to it from a theological perspective in the final chapter, which attempts to describe 'The Politics of Love'.

(4) *Love and transcendence*

Finally we must note the problems created by Halmos' insistence on antinomy or paradox in 'the faith of the counsellors'. Undoubtedly he has succeeded in identifying the value-laden character of professional work. Professional interventions in people's lives are based on certain assumptions about what constitutes happiness, health, adjustment or maturity. Such assumptions cannot be 'proved', and there is considerable danger that the professional's assumptions about what is best for the client will be different from the client's.[28]

Thus the question of the character of the care offered is crucial, otherwise the vulnerability of the client may well be abused. But it is not a justification of professional care merely to say that it is paradoxical, as though this puts it beyond critical scrutiny. (Halmos quotes the theological tag, *credo quia absurdum*, but few theologians would seriously claim that absurdity *alone* justifies a religious belief!)

Faith depends upon insight or revelation which allows us to grasp that which is beyond reason. The absurdity of faith is not that it commits us to irrationality but that it leads to a trust in aspects of reality which reason cannot encompass. It is risky and elusive, but rarely palpably nonsensical. To have faith in love's triumph therefore requires some kind of expansion of awareness which can glimpse a future hope, despite the apparent selfishness and mutual destructiveness of most human actions in the present. Love becomes transcendent when it is suffused with such non-rational hope.

Throughout this book I shall be trying to sketch in this transcendent element, largely through the use of imaginative associations which arise from the day-to-day exercise of professional care. This pointing to the transcendent character of love must, in my understanding, remain tentative if it is to open the vision of practitioners who may not share my religious beliefs. I am not interested in presenting a theology of professional care based on dogmatic certainties. Rather I hope to communicate with anyone who senses the ambiguities implicit in professional work. Thus this chapter may fittingly end where it began, with the fragile imagery of Eliot's poetry.

4. TO CARE AND NOT TO CARE

Ash Wednesday is, as Helen Gardner has observed: '. . . the most obscure of Mr Eliot's poems, and the most at the mercy of the temperament and beliefs of the individual reader'.[29] Perhaps I may turn this obscurity to my own ends, seeing in the poet's words a description of the transcendent love in professional care. To do this is to move the poetry into a context far removed from Eliot's intentions. Yet, at the same time, the tensions which the poem conveys are universal in character and seem to fit well that uncertain status of modern professional work, caught as it is between a religious concept of vocation and a secular understanding of professional power and self-interest.

The petition 'teach us to care and not to care' occurs twice in *Ash Wednesday*, towards the end of the first of the six poems and towards the end of the last. The first poem is notably penitential in tone, reflecting on remorse, on loss of power and on lack of will. It is important to care, yet care too could be misplaced, a futile and a false concern. The sentiment is expressed well later by Eliot, in his *Four Quartets*:

I said to my soul, be still, and wait without hope
For hope would be hope for the wrong thing; wait without love
For love would be love of the wrong thing; there is yet faith
But the faith and the love and the hope are all in the waiting.[30]

The final poem in the *Ash Wednesday* series returns to the penitential theme, but in a new mood. Now there is less to regret, more to give hope. If only we do not 'mock ourselves with falsehood', there *is* hope in the tension within which we live, 'the time of tension between dying and birth'. In the stillness which is neither excessive concern nor hopeless apathy there is a beauty and a oneness to be found 'even among these rocks. Our peace in His will.'

I want to avoid prosaic 'explanations' of Eliot's poetry. This would be the surest guarantee of a loss of all its subtle meaning. But I hope I have been able to convey sufficiently the atmosphere of this poem, to allow its relationship to professional care to be seen. I am suggesting that professional care is one possible response to the fragmentation of our world, which expresses itself in illness and many other forms of social distress. The person who offers professional care seeks (perhaps unknowingly) to restore that lost unity, yet also inevitably shares in the fragmentation. Penitence, hope, realism and a search for a lost harmony are all appropriate and necessary attitudes for people who aspire to care. Eliot's visions convey them all.

An illustration of what I mean may be taken from social work literature. In *Social Work with Undervalued Groups* Ruth Wilkes, protesting vehemently against 'an all-pervasive managerial type of casework aimed at producing results',[31] offers some suggestions about the basic orientation required by those who make it their occupation to help others. She writes:

> . . . it is an approach that calls for humility, patience, an attitude of respect towards the world, and an awareness of its infinite mystery and complexity. This way of helping is difficult because it requires a detachment that does not come naturally. The inclination in any relationship is always to meddle . . . If, however, we can detach ourselves from other people in an attitude of non-possessive concern, we leave them free to change in their own way . . . They are separate beings linked to others through the eye of imagination . . .[32]

We might well regard Wilkes' statements as a commentary on Eliot's words, 'Teach us to sit still'. But is there really hope here, or are we merely indulging in a heady idealism far removed from the realities of professional practice? That is the question which will occupy us for the rest of this book.

TWO

Medical Power

. . . we regard medicine as the most scientific of the
humanities and the most humane of the sciences.

E.D. Pellegrino and D.S. Thomasma[1]

Suffering is only marginally more tolerable when inflicted
with the best of intentions, and the death of Charles II
under treatment by his doctors was much more cruel than
that of his father at the hands of his executioner.

Thomas McKeown[2]

To ward off disease or recover health, man as a rule finds
it easier to depend on healers than to attempt the more
difficult task of living wisely.

René Dubos[3]

We come first to what is indisputably the most powerful of the
'caring professions'. To speak of the power of medicine is to
view it at once idealistically and cynically. In an ideal sense
modern medicine seems to be achieving the conquest of disease
and disability by a remarkable expansion of medical science and
technology. Science may seem to be giving doctors a divine
power, the power of life and death itself. More cynically,
however, we can view medical power as the successful
dominance of the health care scene by one profession whose
claim to effectiveness is in truth poorly founded. The medical
profession above all may seem to invite the radical critique of
professionalism to which I have already referred. The opening
sections of this chapter will attempt to evaluate these
contrasting views of medicine. This will prepare the ground for
a discussion of the doctor–patient relationship in ethical and
theological perspective.

17

1. MEDICAL DOMINANCE

The pre-eminent position of the medical profession in modern health care and in modern society generally has been well documented. In terms of income, social status and influence on health-care policy, doctors are in a more powerful position than any other professional group employed in the health services.[4] The scope of medical authority is remarkably wide and it shows little sign of being curtailed despite doubts about its appropriateness in some instances. The British Abortion Act, for example, allows *any* two registered medical practitioners to authorize an abortion on physical or mental health grounds and *any* other registered practitioner to carry it out. (It is assumed that basic medical training is a sufficient preparation for a procedure with considerable personal and social complexities.) In the field of alcoholism medical facilities for treatment are regarded as appropriate in most countries with a developed health service, even though the aetiology and even the definition of alcoholism remain obscure and the effectiveness of medical treatment uncertain. Medical authority is evident in hospitals for the physically and mentally handicapped, the chronic sick and the dying and yet the major requirement in such facilities is not medical treatment but rehabilitation and humane care. There is also a powerful medical influence in community health care. In Britain the General Medical Practitioner or 'Family Doctor' has been given a 'gate-keeper' role in health care, determining both whether patients are fit for work and whether they should be referred for specialist treatment. This feature of the British health service has been much admired in countries which lack, or have now lost, an effective medical service located in the community. Nevertheless, there is implied a depth of knowledge of the individual patient which may or may not be justified in specific instances, depending on the skilfulness and thoroughness of the consultation which the practitioner offers. Yet his or her authority *qua* practitioner to make such decisions is taken for granted in arrangements for sickness benefit and in the administration of specialist services.

Why has such power accrued to one professional group? Various sociological explanations have been offered. Talcott

Parsons has provided a functionalist analysis which sees the rise to power of the medical profession as a consequence of the increasing division of labour within industrial society. Since illness prevents individuals from performing their social roles effectively, the service provided by doctors is seen as socially valuable. Doctors offer expertise in dealing with illness, combined with an emotionally neutral stance and moral trustworthiness. These qualities lead to the legitimation by society of their authority in matters pertaining to health and illness.[5]

A rather different analysis is provided by Eliot Freidson.[6] Freidson regards medical dominance as a successful political move with considerable rewards in terms of privilege and power. He would agree with Johnson's observation in *Professions and Power* that 'a profession is not an occupation, but a means of controlling an occupation'.[7] The great achievement of the medical profession, in Freidson's analysis, is that it has persuaded governments that it must be granted an exceptionally high degree of autonomy and this has been achieved by successfully established claims to expertise and to 'ethicality'. Freidson's own words on the second claim are perhaps worth quoting in full:

> The profession's service orientation is a public imputation it has successfully won in a process by which its leaders have persuaded society to grant and support its autonomy. Such imputation does not mean that its members more commonly or more intensely subscribe to a service orientation than members of other occupations.[8]

Thus the important difference between the explanation offered by Parsons and that offered by Freidson is that Freidson sees medical dominance solely as a *negotiated* position of power. He does not suggest, as Parsons does, that such a position can be regarded as performing an objectively useful social function. Rather, Freidson uses a conflict model of society, which sees doctors as successful, but not necessarily justified, competitors in a contest for economic and social advantage.

Freidson's analysis depends on assumptions about the egoistic moulding of human nature and society, reminiscent of

19

those of Thomas Hobbes or, indeed Karl Marx and Sigmund Freud. The case he makes has persuasive power, within the limits of his assumptions, but it may not be sufficient in itself to explain the special role of the medical profession throughout history. Of course, even the most fervent admirer of the profession can hardly deny the political manoeuvring and self-interested practices of this, as of every other, professional group. (In this context Freidson's observations on the American Medical Association's approach to medical ethics are instructive.)[9] But it is necessary to explore more fully *why* the medical profession has been granted this very privileged position, and whether we can discern changes in our understanding of health care which could lead to a revaluation of the medical profession's role in society. This will lead us from sociological issues to moral and theological ones.

2. DREAMS, MIRAGES AND HEALTH CARE

In *Health is for People* Michael Wilson has observed: 'Because our model of health is shaped by fear of biological death, cure of disease naturally becomes a supreme value.'[10] Here perhaps lies the secret of medical dominance in modern society. We suppose, rightly or wrongly, that scientific medicine can deliver us from death by removing life-threatening diseases or remedying lethal injuries and disabilities. If this is the foundation on which medical dominance rests then it is a shaky one indeed! We need merely refer to Thomas McKeown's carefully researched survey of the role of scientific medicine in the conquest of disease (*The Role of Medicine: Dream, Mirage or Nemesis*[11]) to discover how little of that conquest is attributable to medical interventions as such. McKeown shows that nutrition, environmental factors and healthy styles of living are the most potent factors in combating disease and preventing premature death. Pharmaceutical and surgical interventions, though not irrelevant or useless, play a relatively minor role. In light of this, McKeown asks why the medical profession have so devalued long-term care in preference to the dramatic cure, when the vast majority of patients seeking medical aid are unlikely to recover.[12]

A slightly different perspective on the same issue is found in

René Dubos' book, *Mirage of Heath*.[13] Dubos attacks modern medicine's concentration on specific aetiology, which he traces back to the success of the germ theory of disease initiated by the discoveries of Pasteur and Koch. In place of the interventionist healer god, Asclepius, Dubos wishes doctors to reinstate Hygieia, the goddess of well-being, consisting of a harmony between mind, body and the natural world. Since in Dubos' view disease is always the outcome of a *constellation* of circumstances (in both the individual and environment), he has a low opinion of the search for 'miracle drugs' and other aspects of heroic medicine. It is pointless to seek for magic bullets to slay the invading disease but to ignore those factors which make the individual receptive to disease. Dubos quotes with approval some words of Francis Bacon: 'The Office of Medicine is but to tune this curious Harp of man's body and to reduce it to Harmony.'

Yet Dubos does not rest content with such musical analogies which invoke only the tranquil goddess Hygieia. He is well aware that harmony is not a sufficient measure of human health, because it ignores an essential human characteristic, the desire to change and adapt to an ever-changing environment. Dubos concedes that in reality there can be no Garden of Eden or Arcadia, where all is at rest: rather, 'to grow in the midst of dangers is the fate of the human race, because it is the law of the spirit'.[14] Thus health must be also defined in terms of the responses to challenges in the (ever evolving) environment. The mirage of perfect health is ever ahead of us and it will never be reached.

We find in Michael Wilson's discussion of health goals (in *Health is for People*) a similar exposition to that of Dubos. Wilson draws a contrast between Adam 'the creature among creatures' and Abraham 'the adventurer moving to unfamiliar places'. Wilson writes: 'Adam flees from stress: Abraham counts the cost and presses onward. Each of us is both Adam and Abraham.'[15] So Wilson resists any simple definition of health, offering instead a whole array of descriptions which might do justice to its complexity and its elusiveness. Wilson stresses that medical treatment is not to be confused with health care. Health care is dependent upon a wide range of services, and more especially upon the quality of our community

21

life. Health 'resents approaches that are too intense'. We may prepare a room for it, as for a welcome guest, but we cannot ensure its presence. It comes unexpectedly, a gift, a grace.

The wider perspective on health which we have now gained inevitably leads to a revaluation of the profession of medicine. The central importance given to the profession within modern health care cannot be justified by any simple appeal to effectiveness, not even if we limit effectiveness to the conquest of lethal disease. We are led to a conclusion very like that reached by Philip Rhodes (himself a medical practitioner) in *The Value of Medicine*: '[medicine] has much more to do with the quality of life than its quantity. It is not a necessity for Man; it is a gloss on his civilisation.'[16]

Why then should this 'gloss' be seen as even at all desirable or valuable? I wish to suggest that the practice of medicine may be seen also in a positive light, but only if the relationship between doctor and patient is radically reassessed. Its potentially health-enhancing nature is all too easily destroyed by the inappropriate expectations of patients and by the false pretensions of doctors.

3. THE DOCTOR AS GOD AND AS BROTHER

My heading for this section is taken from an ancient source – the Hymn of Serapion to the god of healing, Asclepius. The Hymn, which dates to early in the third century AD (and which was reconstructed from fragments in an Athenian museum earlier this century), illustrates well that the ascription of high authority to medical practitioners is by no means a new development. After describing some of the duties of the physician the poem declares: 'He would be like God, saviour equally of slaves, of paupers, of rich men, of princes, and to all a brother . . . For we are all brothers.'[17] A commentator on the poem remarks that such ascriptions of divinity are a 'commonplace' in ancient writings on medicine, while the reference to brotherhood shows the influence of Stoic ideals.[18] No doubt this is so, but the juxtaposition of godlikeness and brotherliness retains a significance for today also, making the quotation strangely apposite. It seems that both the profession and the 'lay public' remain quite undecided between these two roles for

22

the doctor – the loving brother or the godlike saviour. Moreover, the exclusively male language in which the doctor's roles are described remains an accurate reflection of attitudes. Despite the entry of women to the profession, doctors are still viewed as 'gods and brothers', rarely (if ever) as 'goddesses and sisters'. By looking critically at these attributions of godlikeness and brotherliness we may hope to find a more realistic and appropriate understanding of the medical relationship and the place of medicine in health care.

Godlikeness

As one might expect, Bernard Shaw has some sharp things to say about the godlike aura surrounding the medical profession. Among his suggested reforms of medicine he included a requirement by law that doctors have inscribed on their brass plate: 'Remember I too am mortal!' Yet he also observed that blind trust in doctors seemed inevitable so long as people are unwilling to face the truth about the effectiveness of medical treatment.[19] People want their doctors to have godlike knowledge and powers and so they frequently collude in the maintenance of medical dominance. Leo Tolstoy cleverly portrays this in his short story, *The Death of Ivan Ilyich*. When Ilyich consults a doctor, he readily spots the professional manner, so similar to the one which he, as a judge, often used in court:

> . . . The whole procedure followed the lines he expected it would: everything was as it always is. There was the usual period in the waiting-room and the important manner assumed by the doctor – he was familiar with that air of professional dignity: he adopted it himself in court – and the sounding and listening and questions that called for answers that were foregone conclusions and obviously unnecessary, and the weighty look which implied, You just leave it all to us, and we'll arrange matters – we know all about it and can see to it in exactly the same way as we would for any other man. The entire procedure was just the same as in the Law Courts. The airs that he put on in court for the benefit of the prisoner at the bar, the doctor now put on for him . . .

But, despite his clear perception of his doctor's professional tricks, Ivan Ilyich made no real attempt to break through to an honest discussion:

> . . . from the doctor's summing up Ivan Ilyich concluded that things looked bad, but that for the doctor, and most likely for everybody else, it was a matter of indifference, though for him it was bad. And this conclusion struck him painfully, arousing in him a great feeling of pity for himself, and of bitterness towards the doctor who could be unconcerned about a matter of such importance.
>
> But he said nothing. He rose, placed the doctor's fee on the table and remarked with a sigh, 'We sick people no doubt often put inappropriate questions. But tell me, in general, is this complaint dangerous or not?'
>
> The doctor regarded him sternly over his spectacles with one eye, as though to say, 'Prisoner at the bar, if you will not keep to the questions put to you, I shall be obliged to have you removed from the court.'
>
> 'I have already told you what I consider necessary and proper,' said the doctor. 'The analysis may show something more.' And the doctor bowed.[20]

In his humble submission to medical authority Ilyich is merely following the long-recognized correct mode of behaviour for patients. The Hippocratic writings instruct physicians to be servants of their art of combating disease and specify the patient's place as merely to co-operate with the physician in this combat.[21] Nearer our own time, we find an eighteenth-century manual of clinical medicine instructing doctors: 'Make yourself master of your patients and their affections . . . not as a cruel tyrant reigns over his slaves, but as a kind father who watches over the destiny of his children.'[22] In the nineteenth century the Code of Ethics of the American Medical Association recommended a combination of 'tenderness with firmness, and condescension with authority' in order to inspire patients with confidence.[23]

Knowledge is power

If medicine has such a minor role to play in the enhancement of health, what is the use of all this godlike paternalism and authority? An answer may be found in the realization that *knowledge is power*. From earliest times the doctor has been revered because he possesses, or claims to possess, an understanding of health and disease greater than that of his patients. (I use the masculine pronoun deliberately.) In the classical era this was seen as an acquaintance with the healing power of nature and a knowledge of where the force of necessity made cure impossible. The medieval synthesis of medicine and theology gave the doctor a priest-like authority, since illness had always to be understood in relation to the healing of the sacraments and to the patient's eternal destiny. Doctor and priest alike knew better than the patient where health and benefit lay. In our own era the rise of the scientific method has brought a different kind of power. Now we regard the doctor as the person who will save us from superstition and the hazards of ignorance by putting us in touch with the 'scientific facts' of our illness and its possible cure. In his remarkable book, *The Birth of the Clinic*, Michel Foucault describes the emergence of clinical medicine as the advent of a new kind of medical 'gaze' (*regard*) which 'sees' the disease beneath the visible surface of the human body. The scientific doctor has a special knowledge gained from the reading of clinical signs, whose meaning has been discovered by the science of pathology. Thus death has illuminated life. Foucault quotes the nineteenth-century pathologist, Bichat: 'Open up a few corpses: you will dissipate at once the darkness that observation alone could not dissipate.'[24] Foucault comments, '. . . the whole dark underside of disease came to light, at the same time illuminating and eliminating itself like night'.[25]

We are recovering only with difficulty from the remarkable effect of the brightness which Foucault describes so poetically. Dazzled by science, we falsely ascribe to the doctor–scientist a power far greater than that which he or she possesses. We forget that the genuine power of medicine stems from its capacity to identify and co-operate with healing forces already present in the individual, social group and the environment. Medical power depends upon knowledge and skill, but a knowledge and skill which must itself be constantly altering to a wider vision. The doctor and theologian Robert Lambourne described a 'concepts map of disease and deliverance', and he convincingly charted on this 'map' the narrow scope of medical interventions, especially since the scientific revolution in medical care. He saw the error of medicine as its tendency to concentrate on a 'bad focus in the flesh', to ignore a wide range of factors relevant to health, most especially the socio-political dimensions. In an essay published shortly after his death[26] he advocated an 'adaptable catholicity' in both medicine and theology.

The authority of the doctor rests upon this adaptability, which uses the scientific outlook to criticize the false certainties of a narrowly conceived science. The paternalistic claim to an unquestioned authority in health matters (which, as we have seen, patients frequently encourage) must be discarded if the true power of medicine is to be found. That power is found when the doctor genuinely listens to the patient and to the message of the illness and tries to transcend the limits of all previous understanding. It is the doctor as learner who carries a special authority, not the doctor as dogmatist. In *The Voice of Illness*, Aarne Siirala expresses this well:

> Experiences in therapy show that every man becomes sick and healthy in his own individual way. Every human organism cuts its own path to death and life . . . If the therapist tries in his encounter with illness to follow some specific theory of human nature or to cast the sick person in the mould of a certain 'real man', he becomes deaf to the message of illness in the structure of human existence.[27]

Thus the doctor who aspires to (or is pushed toward) godlikeness would do well to seek a more genuine authority in 'brotherliness'. Anne Sexton says it all neatly in these lines from a little poem called 'Doctors':

> They are not Gods
> though they would like to be;
> they are only a human
> trying to fix up a human
> . . .

The doctors should fear arrogance
more than cardiac arrest.
If they are too proud,
and some are,
then they leave home on horseback
but God returns them on foot.[28]

Brotherliness

The fellow humanity of the doctor should open the way for an appropriate use of what limited power is available from medical knowledge and skill. In this context, a quotation from the Hippocratic *Precepts* is frequently cited: 'Where there is love of man (*philanthropia*) there is also love of the art (*philotechnia*).' P. Lain Entralgo, in his short history of the doctor-patient relationship, explains[29] what this means in terms of the Greek philosophy of the time: 'a love for the perfection of the human race as individualized in the patient's body . . . a joyfully reverent love for everything that is beautiful in nature . . . or conducive to beauty.'[30] We should notice that such love does not necessarily give value to the *individual patient*, except to the extent that the individual body *may* participate in a higher beauty. Thus some patients may be more valuable in this respect than others and some, if incapable of restoration of health, are better left alone. (The class distinctions in Greek medicine are clearly portrayed in Plato's *Laws*. The slave doctors, we learn, 'never talk to their patients individually, or let them talk about their own individual complaints', but the doctor who treats the rich freemen 'enters into discourse with the patient and with his friends, and is at once getting information from the sick man, and also instructing him as far as he is able'.[31])

We see a tension between different kinds of love in this conjuction of 'love of man' with 'love of the art'. Every medical art, from the cutting of the surgeon's knife to the interview technique of the psychiatrist may be 'erotic' in character, not in the sexual sense with which this word is often associated, but in the sense of a drive toward that which gives the individual gratification of many different kinds. Doctors may work like artists who seek to make something of the 'material' which is before them; they may value patients as 'good cases', which will help them satisfy the intellectual curiosity which led to choosing a particular medical speciality; or they may find in the successful case and the grateful patient a reassurance that what they are doing has value. Such personal investment gives a dynamism to medical work, but can also lead to the godlike domination which turns medicine into a form of idolatry. To avoid this the doctor must also get close to the individuality of the patient through an awareness of fellow humanity and of mutual dependence. This is the love which is appropriately described as 'brotherly' and 'sisterly', a love which fosters friendship (*philia*). The power of medicine then becomes the power of *letting go* control, using knowledge of the limitations of medical work to encourage the patient to take part in the shared task of trying to understand and deal with the illness as it affects his or her personal being. The doctor as God must be replaced by the fallible human being whose knowledge is incomplete and whose will is corruptible.

Patients, as much as doctors, struggle against such a revaluation of medicine, since it leaves them where they truly are, still vulnerable, still mortal. Yet there is a more solid kind of hope in such a relationship than that which medical idolatry offers. This hope we may now explore in a preliminary way, in preparation for a fuller exposition later in the book.

4. HOPE AND HUBRIS

In *A Philosophical Basis of Medical Practice*, Pellegrino and Thomasma offer the following definition of the medical relationship, 'a relation of mutual consent to effect individualized well-being by working in, with and through the body'.[32] This is a good definition, in the sense that it both delimits and offers an essential identifying characteristic. The limits are set in terms of consent, well-being and individuality. The reference to the bodies of both doctor and patient identifies the unique feature of medical acts as bodily relationships. Medicine deals with embodiments of distress (including those which are found in mental and emotional forms, yet still embodied in an individual life), and it deals with it by means of the body – by vision, hearing, touch. Medicine is not *only* physical, but it is *in essence* physical. When the body is lost sight of, medicine becomes some other activity – counselling perhaps, or preaching. Medicine's contribution to health may be described as an 'incarnation of knowledge' for each individual body. We can see three forms in which the medical relationship offers incarnate knowledge: in *bodily integrity*, in *restoring the stranger* and in *science as prophecy*.

(1) *Bodily integrity*. The first achievement of the development of scientific medicine is its revelation of the secrets of the human body. Though still mysterious in its complexity, bodily existence is more fully understood than ever before. The body has come closer to us, can be owned more fully by us. Medicine delivers us from fear of the body by helping us to understand why it causes us pain and crippling anxiety. The 'doctor as brother' (and as 'sister') educates patients about their own bodies, enlisting them as partners in the attempt to restore control of, and trust in, their organism and its environment. The ritual of the traditional clinical teaching round, in which the 'sacred brotherhood' of doctors and trainee doctors is given privileged access to an understanding from which the patient is excluded denies wholly this hope in medicine. Concealing medical knowledge from people makes them into captives in a bodily prison, trapped in a strange place full of menace, half real, half imagined. However pathological the body's state, such imagined terror is worse and more destructive than the knowledge which is carefully shared. It is reverence for the body, including the damaged and the dying body, which can unite patient and doctor in a common love, a seeking for bodily integrity, however fragile, and however impermanent it may be.

(2) *Restoring the stranger*. In addition to opening the body's mysteries, medicine attempts to explore every corner of the menacing world of illness. The many specialisms in medicine can be viewed as efforts to 'restore the stranger' by extending love and understanding to human situations which are frequently misunderstood or neglected. The old name for the psychiatrist, the 'alienist', conveys this point well. The alienist

worked with those who were feared, or laughed at, or persecuted, because of their differentness, but the chief therapeutic aim of modern psychiatry is to restore the mentally ill to the human community. To a greater or lesser degree, all specialisms in medicine perform similar tasks – geriatrics, pediatrics, the numerous branches of surgery, obstetrics and gynaecology, rheumatology, venereology – whatever specialism is named, there is an area of fear or ignorance which leads to neglect of people's needs and a range of special disability which requires appropriate help. Medical knowledge can and should extend the boundaries of friendship, making the stranger the friend and the unfamiliar a source of learning not of fear. The body of the patient, instead of being hidden from sight as dangerous or unclean, is restored to the human community.

(3) *Science as prophecy*. But although medicine begins with the individual body in its pathology and strangeness, it does not end with the restoration of the individual. Medical advance, as with scientific advance generally, has widespread and powerful social effects, for good and for ill. Medical knowledge reveals the inadequacies of societies; it alters life-styles through spreading awareness of health-risk factors; above all, it raises expectations for health and happiness to previously unimagined heights. (For example dramatic and widely publicized advances in transplant surgery or in human genetics change the whole climate of expectation, to a point where mastery of life and death is sought as of right.)

Thus medicine has a 'prophetic' role, in the sense not simply of prediction of the future (fore-telling) but of warning about the future consequences of present events (forth-telling). There is no possibility of a 'pure' or value-free medical science, which does not commit itself to values. Every medical act and decision promotes some values and neglects others. Siirala expresses this point as follows: 'Every man uses words which are either diabolic or reconciling, corruptive or healing, and the character of his word formation is decisively dependent upon how he encounters the reality of illness.'[33]

Another way of expressing this point is to say that, by virtue of the fact that we give a scientific explanation priority in the encounter with illness, the doctor is granted a prophetic role in modern society. In a phrase coined by Michael Balint, the doctor is given an 'apostolic function' in relation to illness.[34]

The persistence of hubris

It must be said that all three of these incarnations of knowledge are easily neglected in medical practice. Ivan Illich's accusation that Western medicine is guilty of a hubris, which will lead to its own destruction and which is already destroying those dependent on it,[35] may well appear to be closer to reality. The patient and sensitive search for bodily integrity and the consistency required to help restore the stranger are easily swept aside by a *furor therapeuticus*. Doctors tend to have quite infrequent and fleeting contact with the bodies of their patients. Those specialisms in medicine which deal with chronically disabled bodies (geriatrics, psychiatry) are less well esteemed and less popular than those which deal with 'normal people' during episodes of illness which can be cured (surgery, acute medicine, general practice). The wish for cure dominates medicine and the routine tasks of caring are delegated to nurses, who are regarded as more appropriate hourly companions for the patient. We might say that doctors tend to serve the male God of interventionist medicine, Asclepius. The more tranquil, nurturing role of Hygieia, the goddess of well-being, is seen as a lesser task, suitable for the womanly patience of nurses. (I shall explore this stereotype of nursing and of womanhood in the next chapter.)

The neglect of care and rehabilitation leads to a muting of the prophetic voice in medicine. So long as success can be claimed for technological ingenuity there is no need to confront the darker sides of human life, which created the need for such interventions in the first stage. Yet it is the scientific honesty of medicine which should reveal its own inadequacies and the inadequacies of the societies in which it is practised. If eyes are lifted from contemplation of the lesion, pathological organ or incident of illness, questions of causation and of epidemiology are inescapable. The accident–emergency department, the cardiac surgery operation list, the venereal diseases clinic are merely the obvious examples. The maldistribution of resources, the connections between ill-health and poverty, the destructive effects of urbanization, the morbidity arising from unemployment – these and countless more factors, are uncovered simply by the practice of medicine.

The encounter with illness leads to prophecy, but only if there are those in medicine with the courage to challenge the society which gives them employment. Since doctors in most societies are in a relatively wealthy and privileged position, the role of social critic or prophet entails an attack on their own security – hardly something they are likely to welcome! Yet the most important embodiment of medical knowledge is its effect on the restructuring of society in a way which will prevent illness and promote health. The contemporary equivalents of the public health movements and immunization campaigns of the nineteenth and early twentieth centuries are as yet only dimly discernible.

Knowledge, power and love

My aim in this chapter has been to sketch some features of the profession of medicine which might justify the view that in place of medical dominance and paternalism there could be a 'brotherly' (and 'sisterly') love. The secret of medical dominance is knowledge (or at least the imputation of knowledge). I have been suggesting that medical knowledge, when incarnated in individual and society, can serve the purposes of love, in the sense that it can overcome fear, hostility and ignorance, and it can open a path to the enhancement of human well-being in a non-discriminating manner. In terms which will become more familiar as this book progresses, I regard medical knowledge as serving both *philia* (friendship based on mutual understanding and respect) and *agape* (concern for all humankind).

Yet the position of the medical profession will probably always remain a socially dominant one. It deals in an area so close to human vulnerability and finitude, that however modest and well-intentioned its practitioners, an aura of special influence tends to surround them. As a result, there always remains the danger that 'godlikeness' will obscure the limitations of medical practitioners and dependence will prevent people from attempting what Dubos describes as 'the more difficult task of living wisely'. We shall explore in the next chapter the possibility that the nursing profession could more effectively promote such self-reliance.

THREE

Nursing, Nurturing and Sexism

There is no higher mission in life than nursing God's poor. In so doing, a woman may not reach the ideals of her soul; fall short of the ideals of her head, but she will satiate those longings in her heart from which no woman can escape.

Sir William Osler[1]

Doctoring and nursing arose as complementary functions, and the society which defined nursing as 'feminine' could readily see doctoring as intrinsically 'masculine'. If the nurse was idealized Woman, the doctor was idealized Man . . . Her tenderness and innate spirituality were out of place in the harsh, linear world of science. His decisiveness and curiosity made him unfit for long hours of patient nurturing.

B. Ehrenreich and D. English[2]

How can the pay of nurses be kept so low in view of their hours and the nature of their work? Presumably there is an invisible remuneration – the right to act sympathetically.

Ian D. Suttie, 'The "Taboo" on Tenderness'[3]

What is the nature of the care offered in professional nursing? Is it essentially 'feminine' in character? Does it provide a form of health enhancement which 'godlike' medicine overlooks? The word 'nurse' derives from a Latin root referring to nurturing or feeding (*nutrire*, *nutricia*) and it has immediate associations with the suckling of the child at the mother's breast. We seem to be coming very close to the body (from which, as we saw in the previous chapter, medicine tends to shy

34

away) and to a human relationship which is rich in emotion and in mutuality, since child and mother alike gain and give pleasure at the breast. Yet precisely here we also see the dangers and the difficulties ahead. The nurse is *not* the patient's mother and to see her as such is to demean the patient. Moreover, although I shall be using the customary 'she' in referring to the nurse, the sexual stereotyping which this exemplifies must be radically questioned. We shall understand the character of nursing care only when we free ourselves from the traps which sentimentality and sexism constantly set in our path. In particular, we must divest nursing of two sexual stereotypes: the nurse as the doctor's 'handmaiden' and the nurse as the patient's 'angel of mercy'. In place of these stereotypes, I shall be considering the tension in caring between 'being with' and 'doing to', and will then explore the possibility that nursing offers a love which is 'skilled companionship'.

1. SEXUAL ESTRANGEMENT

Sexual stereotyping is a major obstacle to the exercise of professional care within medicine and nursing. Sexuality inevitably affects the close relationships which doctors and nurses have with patient's bodies (as well as entering to a lesser extent into the social worker's involvement with people's personal distress). Perhaps because of these highly charged professional relationships, sexism frequently distorts inter-professional relationships. Tensions between professions are seen in terms of rivalry between the sexes and prejudices are expressed in caricatures of the other gender group – for example, 'emotional women' versus 'heartless men'. Sexist attitudes may be seen as virulent form of discrimination because (like racism) the individuality of a whole class of people is disregarded and they are dealt with in terms of alleged inferiorities which are seen as immutable and as true of all members of the stigmatized group. Sexism equates sexual differentiation with other differences which have no connection with sexuality as such and, on these grounds, justifies discriminatory treatment.

The recent history of the nursing and medical professions

contains several examples of sexual discrimination, some against females, some against males. The most commonly recognized form of sexism is that exemplified in my opening quotations: Nursing is regarded as an occupation especially suited to women because of certain inherent qualities which fit them for this 'feminine' pursuit rather than the 'masculine' pursuit of medicine. Moreover, such stereotyping also regards the nurse as 'naturally' subservient to the doctor, just as woman is 'naturally' subservient to man. This is how an article in a popular magazine published in 1871 sought to attract young ladies into a nursing career:

> . . . here is an opportunity for showing how a woman's work may complement man's in the true order of nature. Where does the character of the 'helpmeet' come out so strikingly as in the sick room, where the quick eye, the soft hand, the light step, and the ready ear, second the wisdom of the physician, and execute his behests better than he himself could have imagined?[4]

Males have also suffered from discrimination if they chose to follow a nursing career in the atmosphere of feminine dedication encouraged by the Nightingale reforms. Abel-Smith describes the negotiations carried out to secure the state registration of nurses as 'rampant snobbery and militant feminism'.[5] Men were placed on a separate register by the 1919 Nurses Registration Act; they could not enter the training schools attached to the major voluntary hospitals; and they were excluded from the College of Nursing. Even today men in general nursing may be regarded with some suspicion, doubts being cast on their masculinity or on their motives for entering the profession.[6] (Curiously, females in medical careers are never thought to be Lesbian or to have illicit sexual motives for entering medicine.)

Are there any logical grounds for such type-casting according to sex? Perhaps women are more naturally suited to nursing than to medicine and perhaps the reverse is true of men. Perhaps, too, nursing should be in a subservient role to medicine and perhaps such a role is appropriately a woman's place in life. To prove any of these assertions we would have to show (first) that there were differences of aptitude or inclination between people, which were due *solely* to their gender differences, not to other factors such as environment, educational opportunity or socially acquired attitudes; and in addition that these differences corresponded to the differences in aptitude and inclinations required for medicine and nursing. Secondly, we would have to demonstrate that all the competence which nurses possess by virtue of their training and experience is of use only so far as it enables doctors' treatment instructions to be followed.

So far as differences in aptitude and inclination between the sexes are concerned, a substantial body of research has yielded very few positive results.[7] Apparent differences may be summarized as follows: males are somewhat better at spatial orientation and females at verbalization; males are more physically aggressive (but not necessarily more verbally aggressive); females are more anxious and less confident in themselves than males; both sexes are capable of empathizing with the distress of others, but females appear to be more willing to do so than males and they show greater interest in the emotional responses of others. These results certainly do not justify broad generalizations about typically male and typically female occupations. They may provide some explanation about why the close contact with patients entailed in nursing is favoured by women, but the research suggests that men are no less *capable* of such closeness. Conversely, nothing in these findings indicates that women are less suited to be doctors than men. However, the lower confidence and aggressiveness of women could provide an explanation of why women as a whole find difficulty in gaining high status positions such as medical consultant, judge or senior business executive.[8] But women's difficulties in pursuing careers are as much attributable to social expectations, educational opportunity and domestic commitments as to the lack of any 'innate' drive to succeed.

What about the subordination of nurses to doctors? The question of whether nursing is to be viewed as a separate profession or merely as a subordinate division of medicine is one which will reappear in various forms throughout this chapter. But even if nursing were rightly entirely under medical authority, it is not clear why, except for the accidents of history, this should be equated with an authority of men over women. Judgements about 'natural' male superiority have no basis in fact, unless by 'superiority' is meant greater physical strength. (Hardly a reason for granting someone medical responsibility!) As we have already observed, women, with their high verbal facility and their interest in emotional problems, seem at least as likely as men to practise medicine well. In any case, the vastly differing proportions of women in medicine in different countries (25 per cent in Britain, 75 per cent in USSR, 7 per cent in the USA) provide a strong indication that cultural factors, not sexual differences, determine whether males and females are granted medical as well as nursing responsibility.[9] If in some countries female doctors are routinely in charge of units with male nurses, it seems odd to claim that male supremacy is part of the order of things.

Thus, in order to understand the quality of care which nursing provides, it is essential to divest it of these sexual stereotypes. If there are particular personality traits which suit a person for nursing (and, in view of the wide diversity of work within the profession, this too might be questioned) differences in such traits are as likely to be seen *within* the sexes as between them. Moreover, the attitudes and abilities which (because of cultural influences) tend to be associated with one sex or another (e.g. sensitivity, patience in the female: decisiveness, intellectual curiosity in the male) seem to complement each other in important ways. The refusal to 'gender-type' a profession can lead to an enrichment of the ways in which its tasks are seen by both men and women. In this context, the term 'androgeny' has come into use. Patricia Geary Dean writes:

> Nurses have some of the very important skills and traits which have been encouraged in women by socialisation: the ability to show emotions, the development of . . . caring, co-operation, listening skills, and the ability to support others. To be able to add to this some of the positive skills which are usually considered a part of the male role – future orientation and problem solving – would make us much fuller human beings as well as more competent professionals capable of providing better care. Let us move on to androgeny.[10]

But for all one's attempts to show the fallacy of sexism, or to promote an understanding of 'androgeny' there remain attached to the images of nursing some other powerful emotional associations which must be fully appreciated before trying to describe the special quality of nursing care. These arise from the other stereotype referred to earlier – the nurse as 'angel of mercy', and from its darker side, the nurse as custodian of one's body, the domineering woman.

2. ANGEL, MOTHER OR BODY-EXPERT?
Angels of mercy

In their paper 'The Faces of Florence Nightingale' Whittaker and Oleson have commented on the heroic image of nursing which was promoted in the nineteenth-century Nightingale reforms. Florence Nightingale succeeded in embodying both romantic and humanitarian values in her account of the professional nurse. Young ladies were encouraged to make the 'safe sacrifice' of a life devoted to the sick – 'safe' because 'although exposed to blood, sweat and toil, [the nurse] remains ever sweet, dainty and eternally feminine'.[11] Whittaker and Oleson quote some adulatory verses from Henry Longfellow's 'Santa Filomena' ('Holy Florence') to illustrate the point:

> Lo! in that house of misery
> A lady with a lamp I see
> Pass through the glimmering gloom,
> And flit from room to room.
>
> And slow, as in a dream of bliss,
> The speechless sufferer turns to kiss
> Her shadow, as it falls
> Upon the darkening walls . . .
>
> A lady with a lamp shall stand
> In the great history of the land,
> A noble type of good,
> Heroic Womanhood.[12]

A striking aspect of this picture of the nurse is her ethereal, evanescent quality. She 'flits' angelically from place to place. There are no coarse bodies here, no festering wounds, no incontinence, no screams of pain. The grateful, silent patient kisses a passing shadow.

39

Not everyone, however, was as enamoured of the innovations of the 'Lady-with-the-Lamp' as Henry Longfellow. Here is how a medical writer in the *British Medical Journal* of 17 March 1880 saw such ladylike nurse pupils:

> As a mere matter of fact, ladies, as a rule, do not make first-rate nurses; and the reason is obvious. With rare exceptions they are essentially *amateurish*; or, if very much in earnest, they are dominated by some principle or power . . . Ladies take to nursing, as a rule, from slightly morbid motive; they are 'disappointed', or they want something with which to kill *ennui*, or they have religious convictions on the subject; none of which sentiments, we may venture to say, are likely to result in producing good *staying* workers.[13]

One can hardly miss the prejudicial attitudes which underlie this writer's comments. No doubt, like many other doctors of his time, he saw the new breed of nurses as a considerable threat to his authority. The old-style nurse, untrained and drawn from the class which provided domestic servants, was easier for the doctors to control and she had no pretensions about her knowledge of the patient's condition, as the new 'ladies' certainly had. On the other hand, the upper-class heroine, modelled on Miss Nightingale herself, may be far removed from the real needs of patients. The old nurse may have lacked training and perhaps also discipline, but her social class meant that she more readily understood and could communicate with the working-class patients who filled the hospital wards of the time. It is not easy to get close to a ministering angel!

As professionalism of nursing continued through the early decades of this century the stress on ladylikeness was gradually replaced by one on competence and dedication. In some memorable phrases Abel-Smith describes the achievement of State Registration as follows: 'With its military heritage showing in its language, its religious tradition conveyed in its sentiment and its humble ancestry revealed in its uniform, the new profession had come of age.'[14]

Yet to what extent was this a gain in caring for patients? As White points out in her study of Poor Law nursing,[15] when the voluntary hospital nurses became more professionalized they gradually moved away from nursing the poor and incurably sick, leaving a gap to be filled by the poor-law institutions, with their lower proportion of trained staff. Again we see a split between image and human need. The professional nurse may see 'basic nursing tasks' as more suitable for trainees and the untrained. The 'angel', flitting past, is now replaced by the skilled professional, over-trained for the bedside care of patients who need simple care rather than cure.

Mothering

Is then the motherly image better than the 'angel' or professional? Perhaps all that is required in nursing is a kind heart and the ability to understand the patient. Certainly the idea that nursing is a kind of substitute mothering has obvious relevance to the vulnerable state which illness creates in people. An article published in 1905 in the magazine *Hospital*[16] put it simply and graphically: 'Nursing is mothering. Grown-up folks when very sick are all babies.' Yet the dangers of this view become obvious in another sentence from that same article: 'Ability to care for the helpless is women's distinctive nature.' The idea that nursing has parallels with mothering easily becomes the excuse for dismissing nursing as 'women's work' or for failing to see some essential differences between the mother–child and the nurse–patient relationship. We need to look much more carefully at the similarities and differences between professional nursing and mothering.

So far as similarities are concerned, the bodily care which seriously ill or senile patients require – washing, feeding, cleaning away excreta, dealing with pressure sores, providing emotional support and reassurance – seems very like the care which the mother gives her child. Moreover, the trauma of illness or accident and the additional disorientating effects of being removed from one's accustomed routines into the strange world of the hospital can make even less seriously ill patients feel like helpless children in need of comfort and constant attention. The 'nurse as mother' is a warm presence in a frightening world, just as the real mother's cuddling soothes away her baby's fears. Thus the care which the nurse provides is simple and familiar, yet vitally important. The body, which has become a source of such discomfort and fear, is handled both

competently and lovingly. The helplessness of illness can be
very degrading unless such respectful closeness is offered.

But the nurse is *not* the patient's mother and the tender skill
which is required is not something which only women can
provide. (With the advent of the 'working mother' fathers
increasingly share the care of very young babies, perfectly
competently, it would appear.) If the comparison between
mothering and nursing is allowed to go unexamined, the
autonomy of patients quickly suffers. Instead of nursing being
a means of appropriate support at a time of need, it can become
a subtle means of control and the perpetuation of helplessness.
The patient is treated as a baby who can never grow up to any
kind of independence. Such dangers are particularly evident
when the chronically ill are being nursed on a more or less
permanent basis. The picture of Nurse Ratched (the 'Big
Nurse') in Ken Kesey's novel, *One Flew Over the Cuckoo's
Nest*, provides an extreme, but none the less telling, example of
mothering as tyrannical control:

> The Big Nurse tends to get real put out if something keeps her
> outfit from running like a smooth, accurate, precision-made
> machine. The slightest thing messy or out of kilter or in the way
> ties her into a little white knot of tight-smiled fury . . .
> What she dreams of . . . is a place where the schedule is
> unbreakable and all the patients who aren't Outside . . . are wheel-
> chair Chronics with catheter tubes run direct from every pantleg
> to the sewer under the floor.[17]

Against such a picture of maternal domination, we need to
understand the nature of nursing as a relationship which
combines tenderness and care for the body with respect for the
individuality of the patient and a consistent effort to promote
independence and self-maintenance. This is also a form of
mothering, but one which lets go and promotes growth rather
than one which dominates and holds back. Such good
mothering requires the ability to see beyond the apparent
helplessness of patients to their potential for recovery. The
trained nurse, as opposed to the unskilled bedside helper,
should have learned to perceive the needs of patients more
objectively and to define goals for the nursing care which is
offered. Instead of being embroiled uneffectively in a reactive

relationship to patients (the 'little white knot of tight-lipped fury' of Nurse Ratched), the trained nurse should try to offer a relationship which promotes the patient's health, or at least supports the patient's own coping abilities. The knowledge of nursing is knowledge, not just of tasks, but of the day-to-day relationships which can promote well-being among sick and suffering people. Nursing practice, if it is to avoid stereotypes, depends upon the development of carefully articulated theories of the nature of nursing care.

Conceptual frameworks

A valuable emphasis on health enhancement and patients' self-care is found in the writings of two American nurse theorists: Lydia E. Hall and Dorothea E. Orem. Hall describes the nurse as a 'body-expert', but this expertise is put at the service of the patient's increase in self-knowledge and regaining of self-control. The 'nurture' which the nurse provides in seeing to the bodily comfort of patients is one which enables them to grow in awareness of their condition and in knowledge of how they can participate in their recovery. The goal is that through the nurse's *care* patients will be helped to get to the *core* of their problems and this in turn helps to see them through to *cure*.[18]

Dorothea Orem places 'self-care' at the centre of her definitions of what she calls 'the art of nursing'. Nursing is seen as an art because it is 'a creative effort of one human being to help another human being'.[19] Orem distinguishes three types of nursing system which define the respective roles of nurse and patient. (The systems vary according to the condition and needs of the patient):

(1) *The Wholly Compensatory System* is required when the patient's capacities for self-care are temporarily or permanently destroyed. In such situations, 'The nurse helps by acting for and doing for the patient'.[20]

(2) *The Partly Compensatory System* is used when the patient's capacities are restricted to a greater or lesser degree. The nurse both helps patients and helps them to help themselves.

(3) *The Supportive–Educative System* is used with patients who need only guidance, support or teaching to enable them to care for themselves. Here (we might say) the patient is most obviously an agent, rather than a passive recipient of care, and the nurse is an enabler or consultant.

Clearly, both Hall's and Orem's accounts of nursing care have considerable value in dispelling the stereotypes of femininity (in either its 'ministering angel' or its 'mothering' form) which, as we have seen, oppress nurses and patients alike. Their theories (and the many others which have been developed since nursing studies became an academic discipline[21]) give nursing a theoretical base different from that of medicine and at the same time give patients a significant part to play in their own care and recovery. On the other hand, there are dangers in such theoretical formulations, not the least of which is the temptation to wrap up in scientific terminology ideas which are quite simple, perhaps even commonplace. Barbara Stevens has warned of the tendency to 'medical mimicry' in nursing theory. In an effort to show that nursing is as much a 'profession' as medicine, some theorists describe the 'nursing process' by what is really a medical model, with 'patient assessment', 'nursing diagnosis' and 'nursing care plan' running in parallel with the doctor's examination, diagnosis and prescription.[22] Similarly, as Katherine Williams observes, when trained nurses learn to relate technical terminology to their tasks of caring for the patient, they can distance themselves from the humanity and individuality of the person cared for: 'The adult person with an unusable arm and leg, who cannot speak or control his excretions, is conceptualised and categorised as "hemiplegic" . . . "aphasic" [and] "incontinent".'[23] Such descriptions, Williams observes, are far removed from the person's own conception of his helpless state.

The danger described by Williams may apply to all attempts to provide a conceptual framework for nursing, whether or not medical terminology (or a mimicry of medical terminology) is used. It is the familiar problem of closeness and distance which is encountered whenever care is professional, but perhaps it is nowhere more difficult to solve than in nursing. The closeness to the body of the patient seems to make 'theory' a cold and over-intellectual pursuit. Yet without some theory describing the nature of the relationship, the closeness is easily exploited. We must ask how well any theory relates to the actual practice of nursing. In order to explore this question in greater detail we may consider some practical examples, first from a study of nursing practice in the long-stay wards in a large psychiatric hospital,[24] and then from a study of nurses' perceptions of the 'unpopular patient'.[25] These will serve to illustrate what I see as a tension between 'doing to' and 'being with' in nursing care, which some theories seem to overlook.

3. DOING TO AND BEING WITH

In her paper 'Getting through the work' May Clark points out that in wards dealing with elderly patients who cannot be returned to the community, the nursing staff tend to approach their work in terms of 'feeding them and keeping them clean and dry'. The patients are (unintentionally) socialized into dependency and the staff define their work in terms of physical tasks, with terms like 'working hard', 'pulling your weight', 'mucking in', 'getting through it'. Poor facilities and shortage of staff emphasize this aspect of the nurses' perception of their task:

> You can't be in two places at once, which you need to be. A lot of mucking around, tidying up and cleaning. So much so we can't really talk to them. When we do sit down we don't want to talk to them. We want to recover. (Assistant, men's ward)[26]

The relationship to patients is thus primarily one of 'doing to', managing the patients' bodily needs as quickly and effectively as possible:

> It's very heavy. The patients are a dead weight. They've all got to be shaved bar about four. You'd got, say, 36 patients, 28 you had to dress. Got no help at all from them. Had to lift their arms, get the sleeve of their shirts and put their arms through; lug them about. Shave and wash them. (SEN, men's ward)[27]

> A rush job, getting them ready for breakfast. Some were incontinent or immobile – very difficult when short of staff. It comes down to dressing and feeding them when there's not much incontinence. (Student nurse, admission ward)[28]

In this context the descriptions by Hall and Orem of nursing as an aid to patients' self-awareness, self-control and therapeutic self-help seem far removed from reality. Not only is talking with patients a luxury which time rarely permits, but, if the opportunity does arise, the staff feel guilty because they are not 'doing' anything:

> When we are sitting with the patients the doctors see and it looks as if we don't really work hard. They say we haven't anything to do when we are talking and listening.[29]

Moreover, staff used to 'doing things to' patients find it boring to have slack time and be working with patients who have more independence:

> Only one thing, there was plenty of work cleaning and shaving on Lawnswood that time went quicker than on this ward. On this ward you have to keep finding jobs. The patients do most: the time drags. (SEN)[30]

Thus the system which emphasizes the patients as semi-animate objects and the staff as body-minders tends to perpetuate itself. Units of this type are underfinanced and largely staffed with students or untrained staff who cannot be expected to see beyond the immediate horizon of 'getting through the work'. A poem published in the *National Asylum Workers' Union Magazine* in 1912 describes with high emotion the difficulty of the mental nurse's task and the meanness of those who finance it. Things may not have changed so much.

Repulsive work we have to do, and bear obscene abuse,
And undergo a mental strain from which there is no truce. . .

. . . Christian virtues show in caring for the weak;
But of the money that it costs for mercy's sake don't speak.

They say 'The sorrows of these creatures almost make us weep,
And we must ease their sufferings, but we must do it cheap'.[31]

It may seem that I have chosen the most difficult area of nursing to discuss the problem of the nursing relationship. After all, incontinent and senile patients present a considerable challenge to anyone seeking to deal with them at more than a purely physical level, irrespective of the time and facilities available. Yet we find when we move into the more popular and better financed areas of nursing that the relationship problem persists, though in a less obvious way. Barbara Stockwell's study, *The Unpopular Patient*, was carried out in four wards in general hospitals, only one of which specialized in geriatric patients. (The others were general medical wards with a wide variety of cases.)

Stockwell noted that interactions between staff and patients were 'almost always entirely task initiated. Nurses did not approach patients unless they were going to carry out some treatment or provide some service or unless they had some specific information they wanted to collect, and on the whole patients did not approach the nurses unless they had a specific need.'[32] When the tasks were completed the nurses removed themselves from the patient areas.

Thus a similar pattern to that on the long-stay psycho-geriatric ward studied by Clark emerges, with the obvious difference that when the nurses were carrying out tasks they had more time to communicate with the patients. Here, however, Stockwell noted the difference between 'popular patients', who were communicated with readily and often with much good-humoured banter, and 'unpopular patients' who were more often ignored or subtly discriminated against in various ways. Stockwell described the main characteristics of the popular and the unpopular patients as follows: The patients the nurses enjoyed caring for were able to communicate readily with the nurses, knew their names, were able to joke and laugh with them and co-operated in being helped to get well. The patients the nurses least enjoyed caring for grumbled and complained, expressed unhappiness at being in hospital and were thought to be exaggerating their suffering or had conditions which the nurses felt to be inappropriate for treatment in their ward.

Stockwell's findings are hardly surprising. They may be summarized by saying that nurses prefer co-operative patients – a finding substantiated by many other studies.[33] Another way of expressing the nurses' preferences would be to say that they sought task-related relationships with their patients and that they found their tasks most satisfying when these were appreciated by the patients in a personal way. They preferred 'doing to' to 'being with', especially fearing the over-demanding patient; but they enjoyed having a limited friendship with those patients who co-operated. The following example of an unpopular patient illustrates Stockwell's findings well:

> Another patient whom the nurses did not enjoy looking after was a woman very crippled with rheumatoid arthritis. She did not grumble, but she became very cross and sarcastic when frustrated either by being kept waiting for assistance or when a nurse was called away in the middle of doing something for her. She commented to the observer that she was always left until last by the nurses and quoted them as saying when they eventually came to her bed, 'We've come to do the old nuisance now.'[34]

I am not quoting this example to imply that nurses are exceptionally uncaring or deliberately discriminatory. Rather, studies like those of Clark and Stockwell show how nurses become caught up in a system of work which leads them unwittingly to overlook the individuality of all but the most co-operative of patients. The difficulty nurses find in spending any time with the more 'difficult' patients is one which anyone can readily understand. The demanding or dependent person seems to ask of us more than we can reasonably give. The routines of task-related nursing care offer a protection, one which we all need when the demands of caring seem too great. Jean Vanier expresses the risks of caring in these lines:

> Love is the greatest of all risks
> . . . do I dare
> leap into the cool, swirling, living waters
> of loving fidelity?[35]

Barbara Stevens conveys the same sense of risk in a comment on the difficulty of applying existentialist categories of 'encounter' and 'authentic being' to the nursing relationship. '. . . one must ask if the nurse *can* function with "authentic being" in an emotion-laden environment, or whether she might be overwhelmed and stunned into inertia by the constant day-to-day emotional upheavals to which she is subjected.'[36]

The gap between theory and the reality of practice in nursing care must be bridged by discovering fresh imagery for the dedicated caring which the outmoded image of 'ministering angel' sought to portray. Such imagery must retain the humanity of the nurse and must give responsibility to patients for participating in their own recovery, or at least learning to accept that which is irremediable. To meet those requirements I now offer the notion of skilled companionship as the epitome of a nursing care which seeks to promote health.

4. NURSING AS SKILLED COMPANIONSHIP

The Code of Ethics of the Canadian Nurses Association describes caring as 'the central and fundamental focus of nursing'. We have seen throughout this chapter how difficult it is to hold that focus. What is required is an account of nursing which is not caught in sexual stereotypes, which is professional without being distanced and manipulative, which is close to the realities of bodily care, yet also sees the personal potential of the patient, which protects the nurse from overwhelming demands, yet which gives every patient full consideration. In short, to understand nursing correctly we need to understand the tensions implicit in all human acts of care – the 'teach us to care and not to care' of Eliot's *Ash Wednesday*.

A way of understanding the 'loving as caring' which is required in nursing may be found by exploring the concept of companionship. This concept has a number of advantages in respect of the problems we have encountered so far – it describes a closeness which is not sexually stereotyped; it implies movement and change; it expresses mutuality; and it requires commitment, but within defined limits. Elsewhere[37] I have suggested that companionship describes a closeness which is neither sexual union nor deep personal friendship. It is a bodily presence which accompanies the other for a while. The image of the journey springs to mind when we think of the companion. Companionship arises often from a chance meeting and it is terminated when the joint purpose which keeps companions together no longer obtains. The good companion is someone who shares freely, but does not impose, allowing others to make their *own* journey.

Nursing care can be companionship of this kind. Firstly, it is bodily presence, but not specifically sexual. Man or woman may be a good companion to the sick person. The skill of companionship lies in sensing the need of the other person and accommodating oneself to the other's idiosyncrasies. Skilled nursing care depends upon such sensitivity. The body of the other person is handled in a way that overcomes embarrassment and a sense of privacy is left intact. Here is the skill of the geriatric nurse especially, as he or she acts as a companion to the old person in a lost, and often confused, last journey. There may be little that can be said on such a journey, but a good companion gives value to what would be merely bodily and mental degradation simply by being tender and patient.

Secondly, nursing is a companionship which helps the person onward. Whether the destination is recovery or death a companion helps the hardness of the journey. So the good companion looks ahead and encourages when all seems lost. The skill and knowledge of nurses makes them able to see, often better than the patient, how the journey can be accomplished. The greatest destruction of nursing care is evident when routines prevent any change and patients are offered no future, but a state of living death.

Thirdly, the closeness of contact between nurse and patient means a costly mutuality for the nurse. It involves 'being with' not just 'doing to'. Companionship is less than friendship, but it does entail the sharing of risks. Here the 'unpopular' patient presents the greatest challenge to nursing. Who will risk involvement with the demanding and apparently ungrateful patient? Nursing is costly in human resources because it is a constant presence with illness, not merely episodic contact. We have noticed how difficult such presence is to sustain. Nurses seek protection away from the patient when there are no tasks to be done. Yet companionship means staying with the 'difficult' person, at least for a time.

But, finally, the commitment of companionship is a *limited* one. Companions are with one for a while, but they have their own lives to lead too. We have seen the dangers – for both nurse and patient – in the idealized picture of nursing as total dedication. The nurse whose life outside the hospital or sick room has its own richness and satisfaction will offer a less demanding relationship to patients than the nurse whose whole fulfilment must be found in helping the sick. Although it can be painful, parting is an essential element in companionship. The other person journeys on – to life or to death.

Thus in the skilled care which the professional nurse offers there may be discerned a form of love. With either an absence or an excess of professional detachment, this love may be lost. But in the delicately balanced relationship I have described as 'companionship' there is a personal involvement and a giving to the other which transcends skill or technique. At a later stage (chapter 7) we shall explore the theological dimensions of such personal care.

FOUR

The Two Faces of Social Work

. . . inherent in the nature of social work is its vulnerability to distortion either in the direction of psychotherapy or of politics.

Zofia Butrym[1]

Doing case work seems to some like setting out deck chairs for the comfort of a few passengers when everyone on board a sinking ship should be manning the life boats.

Bertha Reynolds[2]

'I thought the welfare worker was going to give me some advice as to whether to stay with my husband or leave him. But she didn't give me any advice at all. I think she expected me to keep coming back and by talking it out I would get over it and everything would be back to normal at home. You know what I mean? She gave me the impression that by talking to somebody, all my troubles would disappear.'

J.E. Mayer and Noel Timms[3]

A new direction in our exploration of professional care is inescapable when we turn from medicine and nursing to social work. The social dimension, implicit but rarely fully faced in medical and nursing care, is a major component in social work theory and practice. In speaking of 'the two faces of social work' I intend to identify something positive in a tension inherent in its nature. The two-faced god, Janus, is god of the portal or gateway, a god who looks both inward and outward. Social work is 'two-faced' in this sense. At the centre of its attention is the individual, but both the inner disturbance of this person and the disrupting effects of the environment may be seen as the valid concern of the social worker. The question which remains unresolved is whether it is really possible (unless one is a mythological figure) to look in two directions at once! Is it possible both to care for the individual and to seek for justice in one's society?

In considering this problem I shall discuss first some definitions of social work which attempt to incorporate both individual and social factors. I shall then explore some critiques of these accounts of social work practice and the possible responses to such critiques. Finally, I shall suggest a way of understanding the nature of social work, in both its personal and political aspects, in terms of 'dimensions of hope'.

1. THE NATURE OF SOCIAL WORK

Unlike the longer established professions, social work does not hold a particularly secure position in public esteem. There is considerable ignorance, or misunderstanding, of what social workers do and a widespread feeling that they deal only with deviants or social misfits. Thus, while people readily identify themselves as possible patients of a doctor or a nurse, they are likely to see help from a social worker as a sign of personal failure. Doubts may also exist about whether social workers really 'do anything'; or whether, what they *do* do, merits the honorific title 'professional'. Moreover, the scope of the social work task seems exceedingly broad, ranging from work with families and young children to work with the disabled and elderly, and from psychiatric social work to work in association with the criminal courts and the prison system.[4] Social workers practise in a wide variety of settings, in hospitals, residential facilities of many kinds, in statutory social-work departments and in numerous voluntary agencies. In view of all this diversity, it is not surprising that the identity of social work seems constantly under question,[5] and definitions (and redefinitions) of its specific tasks abound. Here is how the British Association of Social Workers (BASW) has attempted to explain the uniqueness of the task:

Social work is the purposeful and ethical application of personal skills in interpersonal relationships directed towards enhancing

53

the personal and social functioning of an individual, family, group or neighbourhood, which necessarily involves using evidence obtained from practice to help create a social environment conducive to the well-being of all.[6]

We should note that this definition puts personal and interpersonal factors to the forefront. The social worker uses relationship skills to improve 'personal and social functioning' at a range of levels from individual to neighbourhood. One can see here a determination to move away from the 'welfare worker' image of the social worker, which regards the handing over of material benefits, in cash or kind, as the main task. Social work is seen as the offering of a helping relationship, not the dispensation of charity. But the generality of the BASW definition means that it is unclear what specifically this helping relationship might accomplish. How does one assess 'enhanced functioning'? We find one answer to this in Pincus and Minahan's account of the purpose and task of social work in their text-book, *Social Work Practice: Model and Method*:

> Social work is concerned with the interactions between people and their social environment which affect the ability of people to accomplish their life tasks, alleviate distress, and realise their aspirations and values.[7]

We see in this more specific definition that personal factors are given priority – people's life tasks, distress, or aspirations and values determine what interventions are required; their ability to cope is what must be enhanced. So far as the practice of social work is concerned, Pincus and Minahan have a strong emphasis on bringing about change. They describe the social worker and the agency for which he or she works as the 'change-agent system'. In consultation with those who are seeking help (the 'client system') the social worker identifies those who need to be changed (the 'target system') and those who will work together to bring about change (the 'action system'). On occasion, these systems may all comprise the same people – a couple seeking help with their marriage problems might be both the client system and the target system, and (together with the social worker) they alone might comprise the action system. But in other situations (for example, a voluntary agency seeking to improve relationships in one of its residential homes) client, target and action systems could each comprise a different group of people.

Pincus and Minahan claim that social workers will gain a clearer perspective on their tasks by identifying these four 'systems' and seeing how they must interact in order to effect change. The kinds of changes which may be brought about are: (1) enhancing people's own problem-solving and coping capacities; (2) linking people to resources, services and opportunities; (3) improving the operation of such resources and services; (4) helping to influence national social policies to meet human need more justly and effectively. Thus the changes which are brought about by this approach to social work might be summarized in Lincoln's famous phrases as 'of the people, by the people, for the people', since, despite the talk of 'systems', every system is either an individual person or a group of people, and the changes are changes for the sake of people.[8]

Many other theoretical approaches to social work, apart from that of Pincus and Minahan, might be discussed (for a brief summary of the main theories see Butrym, *The Nature of Social Work*[9]), but this approach is perhaps reasonably representative of the main features of current theory. These features are: a stress on interpersonal or social inter-action; a view of the social worker as change agent; and (in the words of the BASW document) 'a value-base which places respect for each individual person at its centre'.[10]

Such 'mainline' theories are open to criticism from two quite different directions. There are those critics who dislike what they see as an activist and over-interventionist stress, and there are those who demand a more radical approach to social work, one which asks searching questions about the social and political values upon which current practice is based. I shall look at each of these criticisms in turn.

Minimal intervention

In discussing Pincus and Minahan's 'four systems' approach Zofia Butrym comments that, despite its obvious value in clarifying what social work is attempting to do, the emphasis on systems and on change conveys a technological and perhaps even a manipulative atmosphere. Two recent British publications, Nicholas Ragg's *People Not Cases*[11] and Ruth Wilkes' *Social Work with Undervalued Groups*[12] represent fully this kind of reaction. Although these writers approach the issue from quite different philosophical perspectives, they share a common value – minimal intervention, based on a respect for the individual. Wilkes states that, 'The good social worker, like the good doctor, does as little as possible'[13] and she deplores (in a phrase quoted earlier) 'an all-pervasive, managerial type of casework aimed at producing results'.[14] Similarly Ragg argues that, 'A personal approach to social work starts from the client's capacity to act, for it is in action that he constitutes himself the person that he is.'[15] Ragg believes that by adopting terms like 'diagnosis' and 'objectives' social work has created a false inequality between worker and client and is contradicting its claim 'to treat people as people'. Both writers want social workers to develop a more reflective approach, one which helps the client develop individuality. The relationship offered should allow clients to regain a sense of agency, removing obstacles to the paths they themselves choose to follow. In Ragg's terms, people should be helped to 'write their own biographies'.

I shall be returning at the end of this chapter to the style of social work advocated in these writings. Such descriptions have a resemblance to the idea of 'love' which I am trying to identify as a central characteristic of professional care. First, however, the challenge to orthodox theory and practice which comes from proponents of radical social work must be considered.

The radical critique

Such a wide diversity of view is encompassed by the term 'radical social work' that any summary inevitably means an over-simplification. Moreover, the term suffers from the same ambiguities which plague 'social work' itself. The radical critique may simply be offering new methods of doing social work, without questioning the long-term objectives of conventional social work; or it may have a quite different vision of society but one which might be achieved either by conventional methods (like individual casework) or only by radically new methods. I have chosen to simplify this complexity by describing only those approaches which are radical *both* in objectives and in methods. I shall identify the following main points in this thoroughgoing radicalism: (1) the assertion of a collective rather than an individual approach to human values; (2) a critique of capitalism as a source of economic exploitation and of unjust distributions of power in society; (3) a view of conventional social work and of the welfare services generally that sees them as the unwitting allies of the capitalist *status quo*.

(1) We find a statement of the first point in *Radicals in Social Work* by Daphne Statham: 'The radical begins with a rejection of the liberal Kantian view of freedom, and sees both him or herself and fellow human beings achieving freedom and personhood in the context of the collective.'[16] The opposition to Kantian ethics is based on its apparent refusal to take into account the social circumstances of individuals. It is argued that while in *theory* 'respect for persons' may mean that each individual is justly treated, in *practice* the separation of the 'public person' from the 'private person' in this approach to morality gives overwhelming advantage to the powerful and offers no real aid to the weak. The philosophy of minimal interference espoused in the liberal tradition merely leaves the economically and socially privileged free to consolidate and expand their favoured position. For this reason radical theorists insist that the humanitarian aspirations of social work can be realized only through social and political changes which bring about a fundamental redistribution of wealth and power in society. It means a class struggle – but not only to redistribute material benefits – the individualist ethic must be also seen as a 'false consciousness'. Thus for example in *Social Work Practice under Capitalism: A Marxist Approach*, Corrigan and Leonard make it plain that a transformation of *experience* is required to revolutionize society: 'In order to understand and transform the world through practice, not only has action to be collective, but experience has to be collective too.'[17]

(2) In line with this collectivist approach, the current inequalities and injustices in modern Western societies (and elsewhere in the world) are seen to be basically economic in origin. Capitalism, with its monopoly of the means of production by massive business corporations and its exclusive stress on profitability and economic growth, has, it is claimed, no genuine commitment to humanitarian values. Against the power of the profit motive liberal attempts to humanize capitalist society are regarded as naive and ineffective. Jeffrey Galper, in *The Politics of Social Services*, summarizes the consequences of capitalism as follows:

> We produce goods, make investment decisions, and determine the number and nature of jobs . . . on the basis of the criterion of profitability. The consequences are an overabundance of goods that do not add up to a fundamental sense of well-being for most people, an absence of goods that we need but are not profitable to produce, jobs that are destructive to the people who hold them, a national psychology organised round competition and consumption, ecological destruction, and exploitation of large parts of the rest of the world to enable us to maintain our standards of material achievement.[18]

Against this background of economic exploitation, the prime source of the troubles with which social work deals is seen to be societal not personal. Here is how the Case Con Manifesto puts it:

> Case Con believes that the problems of our 'clients' are rooted in the society in which we live, not in supposed individual inadequacies. Until this society, based on private ownership, profit and the needs of a minority ruling class, is replaced by a workers' state, based on the interests of the vast majority of the population, the fundamental causes of social problems will remain.[19]

(3) In this context conventionally organized welfare services are revealed to be a mechanism for preventing a degree of political instability which might threaten the capitalist economy and lead to some fundamental changes in the character of society. The poor and disadvantaged are given some help, but only enough to prevent dangerous dissatisfaction. *Individual*

initiative and assertiveness are rewarded, but not *collective* action for radical change. The helping professions, with their strongly individualistic ethic, are themselves products of the capitalist system and their work merely strengthens and perpetuates the ideology of competitiveness and personal success. Thus, as Galper puts it, '. . . the social services deny, frustrate and undermine the possibilities of human liberation and of a just society, at the same time that they work toward and, in part, achieve greater degrees of human well-being'.[20]

On the basis of this political analysis of social welfare in capitalist society, the radical social-work theorists offer an alternative approach. Here the diversity between various theorists is much greater than in the critique of the existing system, but broadly the approach might be categorized as 'revolution from within'. Radicals accept that in order to practise social work at all they will have to work within the structures which they criticize. Suggesting tactics for working *within* the bureaucracy, Corrigan and Leonard quote the motto 'Float like a butterfly, sting like a bee.'[21] (There are, of course, also experimental organizations which operate *outside* the major voluntary and statutory organizations, but to work only in these contexts would be to have a largely marginal influence.) From their position within organizations the radical social workers seek to alter entirely relationships with both colleagues and clients. Their aim is to create a communal ethic, in which the inequality between professional and client is overcome to a point where, as Statham puts it, '. . . the term "client" would become meaningless'.[22] In dealing with clients they attempt to organize and politicize them in order 'to build a base for radical challenge to the social order as a whole'.[23] This means, as Corrigan and Leonard make clear, a conscious and carefully planned alliance with the 'working class movement'. They write:

> . . . it is not enough to simply join a working-class party and a trade union and work politically within it . . . It becomes vital to discuss the problems of your practice in these institutions, to relate them to working class activists and Marxists, to show the importance of such issues in the overall class struggle.[24]

Perhaps the full implications of this different style of social work are nowhere more obvious than in some of the clauses of the 'Code of Ethics for Radical Social Service Workers', which Galper offers at the conclusion of his book:

6. I will use information gained from my work to facilitate humanistic, revolutionary change in society.

7. I will treat the findings, views and actions of colleagues with the respect due to them. This respect is conditioned by their demonstrated concern for revolutionary values and radical social change.

. . .

14. I will contribute my knowledge, skills, and support to the accomplishment of a humanistic, democratic, communal socialist society.[25]

On the basis of political commitments of this kind, Galper can claim that, 'Radical social work is little more than social work that has not compromised its own commitments to human welfare,'[26] and for Corrigan and Leonard, Marxist social work practice is 'a truly human response to human suffering which confronts an inhuman society'.[27]

2. THE RESPONSE TO RADICALISM

Here then we see one vivid picture of the 'other face' of social work, the face looking outward to society. But the features of that face, as portrayed by the radicals, make it far from acceptable to many social-work theorists and practitioners. Ruth Wilkes' description of it as 'puritanical, joyless and frighteningly dedicated'[28] summarizes a common response from the 'liberal' (whose efforts to reform but not revolutionize capitalist society are regarded as politically useless by the radicals.) The reaction of Paul Halmos (to which I have already briefly referred in chapter 1) is one of the more extreme. He deliberately dichotomizes the political and the personal, thus apparently insulating what he calls the 'personal change-agent' (the social caseworker) from the radical critique. The *political* change-agent is typified as partisan, universalistic, dominant, and dealing with people 'segmentally' (e.g. as 'working-class' or as 'old-age pensioners'): the *personal* change-agent is typified as non-judgemental, interested in uniqueness, stressing mutuality and dealing with people 'globally' (i.e. with their whole personality). In working with people, the personalist is seen as tentative, open to self-criticism, flexible and non-manipulative, while the political activist is characterized as forceful, stressing cognitive certainty, seeking new rules and using people as means to ends, in Machiavellian style.[29] Little wonder then that Halmos, having set up these caricatures, suggests that each of them has much to learn from the other! But what Halmos will not allow is what he calls 'hybridization', that is, any attempt to achieve some synthesis of the personal and the political. Thus, in effect, his response to the radical critique of social work is to accept its polarization (its rejection of any compromise in terms of 'liberal reformism') but to ignore the main brunt of the radical argument, which is that personalism is *also* political, in a conservative rather than a radical manner. Halmos' response is really that of a convinced personalist. He cannot see any real weaknesses in that viewpoint, and he doubts the moral trustworthiness of those who criticize it.

A more helpful response to the radical critique will be one which avoids what Geoffrey Pearson tellingly describes as 'frozen images'.[30] Pearson points out that social work is and always has been caught in an ambiguous relationship to social structure. As he puts it, '. . . on the one hand, it provides an expression of the liberal, humane impulse towards the "good society": on the other, the control of the useless, expendable waste products of the "goods society".'[31] The failure to see this ambiguity results in posing the question of the task of social work in frozen images, like therapy *or* reform, casework *or* revolution. A refusal to allow this dichotomous thinking enables us to see (in Pearson's view) that social work operates at the intersection of what is personal and what is political. It tends to regard people both as autonomous agents and as the victims of socio-political forces.

Following up this insight from Pearson, we may respond to the radical critique by looking more carefully at its argument for political activism in social work. We can see that there are three stages in the argument: (1) a political and moral analysis of capitalist society; (2) an account of how social work currently operates; (3) recommendations about how social work should operate in order to achieve the objectives which the radical theorists regard as desirable. It is possible to accept parts of this analysis without necessarily being committed to the whole.

(1) So far as the political analysis is concerned, it may readily be conceded that capitalism creates inequality and that the criterion of profitability is a poor measure of what will benefit humanity. At this level, the personal and the political must not be polarized. The character of individual life is intimately bound up with the character of social life and this in turn is affected by economic and political factors. Political and economic change is an obviously powerful way of enhancing or degrading the lives of individual persons. Disagreement begins, however, about how such change is to be effected and about whether we have any clear and reliable picture of the kind of society which would be more just and humane than that created by capitalism. Here we see the vital difference between the reformer and the revolutionary. The reformer seeks piecemeal change by persuasion and by the use of inviolable 'democratic means': the revolutionary sees democracy within capitalism as a cloak for the continued advantage of the powerful and aims to subvert the existing order by mobilizing the powerless and disadvantaged to take over control of social institutions. The reformer doubts whether radical change will be for the better; the revolutionary sees no other way of helping the disadvantaged. Eventually (as several writers have pointed out[32]) we find two opposing conceptualizations of social reality: a *consensus* model and a *conflict* model. The former regards the harmonization of competing interests to be possible in a pluralistic society, with inequalities gradually being evened out (or at least mitigated) by common consent or bargaining: the latter sees conflict and gross inequality as inevitable, with a ruling class oppressing a working class and unwilling to change except in response to a greater power. One is left with a decision about which set of basic assumptions is the more convincing.

(2) However, whether a consensus or a conflict model of society is adopted, the radical critique of current social work

practice may prove to be too simplistic. If it is granted that social-work services, operating within a capitalist society, do achieve some amelioration of the living conditions, community facilities, family relationships and personal integration of the socially disadvantaged, then such gains are themselves politically significant. If we take the BASW goal of 'enhanced personal and social functioning' as an example of current social-work aspirations, then we can see social work as an equalizing of opportunity which must create a challenge to the existing distribution of wealth and power, albeit slowly and undramatically. To improve conditions is to create a demand for greater justice. It would not be inconsistent for a person to believe that capitalist society *did* foster injustice, but to use existing social-work provisions as a means of evening out the inequalities. The best resource of the capitalist, then, in order to hold on to advantages, would be to reduce support for conventional welfare services (a trend very obviously developing in the U.K., and elsewhere, at the present time.) In this sense the personal service of social work is also productive of political change, since (as Pearson puts it) it is at the intersection of the personal and the political.

(3) Finally, the radical's recommendations for a new style of social work do not necessarily follow from the previous steps in the argument. Peter Leonard has pointed out that a conflict model of society permits at least three models of what social work does, or might do:[33] (a) The *control model* uses social work as a means of defending the interests of the ruling class. (This is how the radical critique views current practice.) (b) The *adversary model* uses social work to promote revolutionary action, of a non-violent kind, in the interests of the subject class against the ruling class. (This is the role for social work promoted by radical theorists.) But (c) Leonard suggests that at least one more model is possible, the *mediation model*. In this model, social work is given an 'advocacy' role on behalf of the disadvantaged. In addition to offering support to individuals or groups, the social worker recognizes the obligation to organize pressure groups, alert people to their welfare rights and seek to influence legislation. Leonard describes the social worker in this model as tending to have 'a conditional, though

reluctant, commitment to the existing social order'.[34] It would seem that the BASW definition has such a model in view when it states that social work 'necessarily involves using evidence obtained from practice to help create a social environment conducive to the well-being of all'. This statement virtually commits all social workers to some form of specifically political action, but it avoids the conviction of the radicals that only revolutionary social workers have the welfare of mankind genuinely at heart. What the radical analysis does reveal is that it is impossible to have 'non-political' or 'a-political' social work. Social work both proceeds from political policies and has political effects of either a conservative or a transformative nature.

Pace Halmos, then, it seems that we must 'politicise the personal' in social work, but we need not become the Machiavellian revolutionaries of his caricature. It is open to one to accept the greater credibility of the conflict model of society, but to reject the subversive role for social work which some radicals promote on the basis of this model. Love for the individual need not fall into the trap of conservative individualism, and hope for the transformation of society can be 'revolutionary' even when it rejects the use of power. Genuinely to love the individual client is itself to begin to change society. Such 'dimensions of hope' in social work with individuals are the subject of the concluding sections of this chapter.

3. THE PERSONALIST EMPHASIS

Some memorable lines from Yeats' 'The Second Coming' may serve to introduce this section:

> The best lack all conviction
> While the worst are full of passionate intensity.[35]

The problem which confronts us in trying to understand the relationship offered in social work is that (as we saw earlier) there is an absence of agreement both about what social work should be doing and about how it is to be done. The result is a vacuum into which various enthusiasms are sucked, whether for personal counselling, community work or political activism. Parallel to these enthusiasms the 'knowledge base' of social work theory keeps shifting, from psychology to social psychology to sociology to political economy. But perhaps 'the best lack all conviction', since, while social work seeks to find its own identity, the human distress which brought it into being in the first place continues apparently unabated, and 'the best' keep trying to find ways to be helpful, ways to help effectively and without fanaticism.

The hope enshrined in social work is elusive, but none-the-less important. It is a hope for each person in his or her individuality, a refusal to abandon anyone as 'hopeless' or to concede too quickly that destructive forces in society will prevail even in the worst circumstances. The social worker comes empty-handed into situations. There is no physical treatment to try out, no bell, book and candle to exorcize the demon. In social work the relationship must be central, since that is all that there is! Yet it is precisely here that the greatest uncertainty lies. Peter Leonard describes the social work relationship as 'that dreaded idol of traditional social work'.[36] Yet need it be an idol? Need it merely preserve the *status quo* in an unjust society?

We saw how Wilkes and Ragg suggest an answer to such questions in terms of enabling people to live their own lives more fully. Ragg gives the social worker an educational role primarily. The aim is to help through a personal relationship which, because of its sincerity and honesty, improves the client's capacity to characterize his or her own actions and to make rational plans. Self-description becomes a means to assuming a richer identity and to gaining a more confident approach to the problems which oppress the person. Ragg sums up the social casework task as follows: 'It is to teach . . . people how to describe themselves and their situation in such a way as to be able to act as rationally as possible.'[37]

We see in this definition an emphasis on what is sometimes called 'client self-determination'. Since its formulation in Biestek's *The Casework Relationship*,[38] this concept has held a central, if controversial, place in social-casework theory. Many writers have pointed out its ambiguity. Alan Keith-Lucas has identified several possible meanings: client participation in decisions, non-interference with clients except in essentials, clients' rights to accept or reject help offered, and the development of clients' capacities to make their own decisions.[39] It is evident that Ragg's approach is emphasizing the last of these. Others have argued that self-determination has obvious limits, either because it could result in the client causing harm to self or others, or because (in practice) the social worker acts as a controlling influence on the client, with only an appearance of encouraging the client's independence.[40] The latter criticism is well illustrated in the following case described by Wilkes:

> Miss A.T., who was twenty-four years old and mildly spastic, moved from her house in London to the Midlands to work in sheltered employment. She stayed in a hostel attached to the workshop and applied to the local authority for financial help. Well-meaning directives from senior social work staff urged the social worker not to be misled by the problem presented (the request for financial help), but to probe beneath the surface where some deep emotional problem would surely be lurking. The social worker set about Miss A.T. and her parents until he had worked them up to the point where the latter were spending time and money travelling to and from the Midlands for case conferences. Before the web of her emotional life could be officially untangled Miss A.T. left the hostel and ran away with a sailor, presumably taking her deep emotional problem with her.[41]

The problem is how to define social work interventions which are caring, but not meddlesome or manipulative. People who seek assistance may find their problem redefined by those who feel they know better, and attempts may be made to deprive them of a freedom which they had before – a freedom to learn by their own mistakes (if, indeed, Miss A.T.'s action was a mistake). Such a conviction of 'knowing better than the client' is as true of those who seek to 'politicize' clients as it is of those who want to offer them therapy. Both approaches can devalue clients' own perceptions of their lives and of their goals. Self-determination must mean the right to try to achieve something for oneself (and to fail if need be),[42] subject only to the restraints of laws which govern everyone's actions. The fact of being a 'client' should not justify more restriction on action than any citizen may reasonably expect.

The enabling of self-determination (as I have now sought to clarify it) makes social work into an important form of 'loving'. It is the expression of an extraordinary hope – that, given appropriate support and encouragement, people can move from being the victims of circumstances to being those who take control of circumstances, seek to alter them and, by their experience, learn to help other 'victims'. It is obvious that, for much of the time, such hopes are never realized: but the point I have been seeking to establish in this chapter is that only by recognizing the dimensions of hope in social work can we properly understand its nature. It remains for me to explain what I mean by speaking of the 'dimensions' of hope.

4. DIMENSIONS OF HOPE

Like many other over-used terms, 'dimensions' has become debased coinage, with little meaning-value left. Yet it is potentially rich in meaning. To see the dimensions of an entity is to move from a flat, static picture of one aspect of its nature to an understanding which has both depth and movement. To pay attention to the third and fourth dimensions of things is to see at once the poverty of our usual perception. We realize that we see only one or two facets of a solid object, from an angle determined by our view-point and at one moment of what may be a process of gradual or rapid change. Four-dimensional thinking acknowledges the subjectivity of our perception and its proneness to distortion by the accidents of time. If such limitations are true of our perceptions of inanimate objects, they are *a fortiori* true of those complex entities we call 'persons'. We are constantly in danger of a one-dimensional perception which sees no depth and fails to allow for change.

Social work, with its steadfast determination to move from the presentation of a problem to a personal relationship which sets the other person free, provides us with several dimensions of hope. Firstly, it restores the 'problem' to the person, seeking the depth behind the surface presented to one's immediate gaze. In this third dimension the social worker finds hope, assuming that (in some situations at least) the move back to the solidity of personal being is a move to the special knowledge required *for this person* (and no other) to regain control. Secondly, social work places the person in a multi-dimensional environment – a being in complex interaction with an all-surrounding space. Such perception must (as I have argued earlier) lead to social and political action. On the other hand social work is in grave danger of one-dimensionality if it approaches each client with a *prior* picture of what such action will be. The particularity of the client is the starting point. The socio-political action should be hope for *this* person, not for a group to which the individual must conform.

Finally, the time dimension in social work is perhaps its most daring hope. To offer a personal relationship rather than to seek to condition, manipulate or organize others, is to oppose all forms of total determinism with a confidence that time ushers in the genuinely new in the lives of individuals, social groups and even whole societies. Such hope must often look like facile optimism in the face of the tragedies of human history. The Marxist can see such hopes for personal trans-formation as mere illusion, helping to prevent revolutionary change. Certainly it *is* hope, not knowledge. But the hope is also a modest one – that there are some significant changes to be brought about by the simple expedient of helping people to see that the forces which oppress them flourish on *their* lack of hope for themselves. It sets the forces of the individual, not the collective, against injustice. W.H. Auden has a poem of deep despair about modern society entitled 'The Shield of Achilles'. In this poem the harmony and beauty of the ancient world are sharply contrasted with the drabness, inhumanity and apathy of modern society. Here is how the poem ends:

> A ragged urchin, aimless and alone,
>   Loitered about that vacancy, a bird
> Flew up to safety from his well-aimed stone:
>   That girls are raped, that two boys knife a third,
>   Were axioms to him, who'd never heard
> Of any world where promises were kept,
> Or one could weep because another wept.[43]

I have been suggesting that the 'love' of social work dares to add dimensions of hope to that despairing picture, hope that begins where the boy loiters alone. This is certainly not to deny the importance of the political, but it is to prime political change with the dynamic of personal relationships.

FIVE

The Claim to Purity

The regimen I adopt shall be for the benefit of the patients . . .
Pure and holy will I keep my Life and my Art.

Oath of Hippocrates

I solemnly pledge myself before God and in the presence of this assembly to pass my life in purity and to practise my profession faithfully.

Florence Nightingale, *Pledge for Nurses*

Social work . . . requires of its practitioners integrity, compassion, belief in the dignity and worth of human beings, respect for individual differences, a commitment to service and a dedication to truth.

Code of Ethics,
National Association of Social Workers (USA)

Within all the ambiguities and complexities of professional care I have now suggested positive features which may form the basis for love in some form. 'Brotherliness' in medicine, 'companionship' in nursing, 'hopefulness' in social work all imply a commitment to the welfare of others which transcends personal advantage or professional advancement. But is there any basis to the view that such disinterested love is genuine? To this central question we must now turn. The notion of 'vocation' has become rather out-moded and the much quoted accusation by Shaw that professionalism is a conspiracy against the laity seems less outrageous than it might have been when professions kept themselves aloof from strikes and 'industrial action'. Yet the need to trust those who deal with one's body or one's personal problems gives continued force to the hope that there is more to the practice of medicine, nursing and social work, than the pursuit of money and status.

The question of motive cannot be answered by pointing to the presence of dedicated *individuals* within professions. Examples readily spring to mind of people who are so obviously motivated by a sense of commitment that they seem tireless in their efforts to help others. (The moral ambiguity of such commitment, however, will be explored at a later stage – see chapter 7.) It must be with the possible motivation of the professional groups *as a whole* that this chapter is concerned. The question to be explored is at once psychological, ethical and theological: is it possible for a whole group genuinely to profess 'love of neighbour' in activities which are also a means of livelihood and a source of status and influence? How do altruistic and egoistic motives inter-relate in such professional relationships?

1. LOVE, SELF-LOVE AND FELLOW-FEELING

An evaluation of altruism in professional work requires first an analysis of the apparent conflict between love of self and love of others in human conduct generally. The claim to professional dedication, and the critique of it, rest on certain assumptions about the nature of moral agency which must be briefly discussed. In the analysis which follows I shall be relying in part on the ideas of Erich Fromm and Paul Tillich, but most especially on Max Scheler's rich and fascinating work, *The Nature of Sympathy*. (Readers who find theoretical discussions wearisome may wish to turn to the practical applications to professionalism, in the later sections of this chapter.)

Erich Fromm

In several works, notably *Man for Himself* and *The Art of Loving*, Erich Fromm has sought to show an essential complementarity between love of self and love of others. The biblical injunction, 'love your neighbour *as yourself*', is seen by Fromm as an affirmation of the equal importance of care and respect for oneself and for others. Basing his views partly on his experience as a psychoanalyst, Fromm sees selfishness as a *lack*

71

of self-love, since it consists of an anxious grasping for things to compensate for low self-esteem.[1] The person who lacks self-love cannot love others freely and fully. Rather, the relationship is one of symbiosis, in which the needs of the helper dominate the care offered:[2] 'If an individual is able to love productively he loves himself too; if he can only love others he cannot love at all.'[3]

Fromm's account of love also places great stress on what has been referred to in philosophical literature as 'respect for persons' and in theological literature as *agape*.[4] Love, avers Fromm, is not simply an emotional state. It is 'an attitude, an orientation of character, which determines the relatedness of a person to the world as a whole'.[5] This orientation is characterized by 'active concern for the life and growth of that which we love', and it comprises care, respect and responsibility.[6] So in loving both self and others we are not merely responding to the vagaries of feeling: we are taking up an attitude which guides our behaviour consistently and in a unified way.

Fromm's account is interesting and attractive so far as it goes, but it leaves unanswered some fundamental puzzles in the enigma of human loving. Firstly the obvious *lack* of love in human relationships does not seem to be adequately explained (despite Fromm's notable attempts to do so in other works, e.g. *The Fear of Freedom* and *The Anatomy of Human Destructiveness*). Fromm seems insufficiently aware of the brokenness of human relationships and of the pervasive influence of self-seeking motivation. To the theologian, the missing element in Fromm's account is a doctrine of sin (a feature which Fromm himself would see as more of a benefit than a lack, since he regards such doctrines as an unjustified slur on human nature). Another problem in Fromm's account is that the relationship between love and sympathy (or benevolence) is not discussed with any philosophical rigour. Yet this relationship is a crucial one for any moral theory. In Hume's moral philosophy, for example, feelings of sympathy hold a central place: but in Kant's theory such feelings are irrelevant, since they cannot be a matter of obligation. Fromm's psychoanalytical account, despite its important insights into the character of love, seems merely to blur this issue. He denies that love is an emotion but fails to explain

72

adequately how the attitude he is commending is related either to reason or to feeling.

Paul Tillich

In Paul Tillich's writings these neglected aspects in Fromm are usefully discussed. Tillich describes love as power, the power which brings about the union of the separated. Separation is at its most extreme between individual human persons, for, since the centre of such self-conscious individuals is wholly private, they cannot be made mere parts of a higher unity. Thus the greatest power of love is the reunion of individual persons: in Tillich's words, 'The individual person is both the most separated and the bearer of the most powerful love.'[7] Such an account sees love as the most fundamental experience of human life, indeed as the power of life itself. Thus God is appropriately described as love; and love, understood in all its fullness, *is* God.[8]

Like Fromm, Tillich rejects the idea that love is merely an emotion, but on the other hand, he sees the emotional *element* in love to be of central importance. Opposing the radical separation between *eros* and *agape* espoused by some theologians (notably Anders Nygren[9]), Tillich asserts the importance of the passionate element in all loving and sees love, in all its forms, as one. He distinguishes four forms of love – *epithymia* (desire), *eros* (the search for value), *philia* (friendship) and *agape* (the depth of love). Each form, he argues, requires the other three or it becomes distorted. *Agape* is in a special relationship to the rest, since it is the love which is also God, and thus a love which overcomes the ambiguity of the others. But *agape* must not be divorced from the other forms. It participates fully in them 'without losing its eternity and dignity and unconditional validity'.[10]

We find in Tillich some answers to the problem of the failures of love and to the question of how its rational and emotional features are inter-related. Failures in love can be explained by an account of sin as separation. (Elsewhere Tillich uses the term 'estrangement' to describe the separation.) Love is lost, either because the different forms of love become separated and so distorted, or because the estranged character of human individual existence will not yield to the uniting power of love. Very important in Tillich's thought is the continuing *ambiguity* of the human situation. There can be no easy certainty that love will triumph. The optimism we find in Fromm is not evident in Tillich. Rather, faith in the face of deep doubt is needed to believe that love can prevail over estrangement, a faith made possible by the revelation of the New Being in Jesus the Christ, but one which human history seems constantly to threaten. So Tillich speaks of a 'courage to be', in the face of deep anxiety. Only through such courage is loving a genuine possibility.

As regards reason and emotion, Tillich's account of the different forms of love provides an earthing in human desire and emotion but one which enriches Fromm's psychology. Perhaps the greatest of Tillich's contributions is his concept of acceptance, which at once locates love in the most basic of human experiences (as Fromm wishes to do) and yet shows the transcendent element, taking the individual beyond the confines of his or her own security. Acceptance by God creates in us the possibility to accept and love others. Thus Tillich gives theological depth to Fromm's treatment of the egoism/altruism issue by his creative descriptions of the doctrine of sin as estrangement and the doctrine of grace as acceptance.

Yet when all this has been said, there remains a problem which Tillich copes with only in a purely formal way – the problem of the relationship between the transcendent power of *agape* and the more personal forms of love described by *epithymia*, *eros* and *philia*. For, we cannot *feel* the same about everyone. Some people attract us more than others. Some elicit our sympathy: others do not. Yet the demand of *agape* is to love all our neighbours equally and without partiality; and it is precisely this agapeistic regard which is stipulated in professional ethics. In this context, Maimonides' *Prayer of a Physician* is appropriately cited:

> Endow me with strength of heart and mind so that both may be ever ready to serve the rich and the poor, the good and the wicked, friend and enemy.

How is such equal love possible? And what is its relationship to reason and emotion? Here we must turn to Max Scheler's more detailed study, *The Nature of Sympathy*, for a richer answer than we find in either Tillich or Fromm.

Max Scheler

We can most readily understand Scheler's account of love and sympathy if we realize that he was seeking a mediating position between Kantian ethics with its stress on rational obligation alone and the ethics of Hume, Rousseau and the Utilitarians, which (in various ways) gave primacy to desires and feelings. Scheler wished to develop an ethical standpoint which accorded full weight to human feelings, yet which grounded morality in objective values, not merely in emotional reactions. Consequently he undertook a painstaking analysis of the concept of sympathy and of the related concepts 'fellow-feeling' (*Mitgefühl*), 'mutual feeling' (*Miteinanderfühlen*), 'vicarious feeling' (*Nachgefühl*), 'empathy' (*Einfühlung*), and 'identification' (*Einsfühlung*). Scheler saw all of these as relevant to morality, but only to the extent that they prepared the way for love (*Liebe*) which is not a *reaction* (as the others are) but an *action*.

There is a wealth of interesting material in Scheler's discussion of the various sympathetic reactions, much of which is highly relevant to an analysis of professional motivation. Unfortunately only a small sample can be included here. Scheler begins with the fundamental point that all the forms of sympathy are 'blind to value'.[11] For example, we may as easily rejoice in A's pleasure as B's misfortune as feel compassion for B. (The sympathy of a sadist with a fellow-torturer is no less sympathy for being morally deplorable.) Since sympathy is a *reaction*, it is contingent upon our attitudes as a spectator, not upon the value or disvalue of what we observe. Nevertheless, the various forms of sympathy may *lead* to that which is morally good, the exercise of love.

(1) At a basic level we have the phenomena of mutual feeling, vicarious feeling and 'emotional infection' (*Gefühlsansteckung*). Scheler illustrates mutual feeling in a few graphic lines:

> Two parents stand beside the body of a beloved child. They feel in common the 'same' sorrow, the 'same' anguish . . . they feel it

together, in the sense that they feel and experience in common, not only the same value-situation but also the same keenness of emotion in regard to it.[12]

A similar, though less intense, experience is that of vicarious feeling, when, in witnessing the distress or joy of the other, I (to an extent) sense its quality. (Scheler's favourite example here is the terror of a drowning man, which one may resonate to, though the real terror is his.) There is also 'emotional infection', of which abundant examples may be found in crowd behaviour, group hysteria, etc.[13] Here emotions are transmitted from person to person with great force, but without any knowledge of how the other feels. (Of all the phenomena of 'feeling with' this last one is the least voluntary and the most devoid of value-reference.)

(2) Although these three examples are in a sense 'fellow feeling', they lack an element which Scheler sees as essential to sympathy in its fullest sense. Feeling *with* the other demands full participation in that which is other than one's own experience. It requires empathy and (at least to some extent) identification. (The progression is clearer in German – *Einfühlung and Einsfühlung*). Scheler is at pains to stress that such participation, especially at the level of identification, is not deliberate and rational in character, but a letting-go of self, more characteristic of primitive cultures or of the childlike vision, than of modern Western man. (He includes among his examples of emotional identification taking on the characteristics of a totem animal, hypnotism and ecstasy in sexual union.) The loss of the capacity to identify with others and with natural objects is seen by Scheler as a grave defect of modern culture, with a consequent instrumental and dominating view of one's fellow humans and the natural environment.[14] The recovery of the capacity (although itself unconscious and non-rational) could lead to greater efforts to understand others at a rational level. Scheler thus sees such experiences as occupying a mediating position between body and mind:

> To attain identification, man must elevate himself 'heroically' above the body and all its concerns, while becoming *at the same time* 'forgetful', or at least unmindful, of his spiritual individuality;

he must abandon his spiritual dignity and allow his instinctive life to look after itself.[15]

(3) Against this background Scheler introduces his account of the nature of love. He believes he has identified in fellow-feeling '. . . a genuine *out-reaching* and entry into the other person and his individual situation, a true and authentic *transcendence* of one's self'.[16] This alone is enough to prevent naturalistic reductions of altruistic feelings to egoistic ones, so Scheler believes. We reach out to others for motives which cannot be described as self-seeking. Nevertheless such reaching out does not of itself create moral value. It all depends upon what such feelings enable, for, we must recall, they are blind to value. Here love enters in. Love is 'that movement wherein every concrete individual object that possesses value achieves the highest value compatible with its nature and ideal vocation'.[17] Thus we can regard love as in a sense both 'creating' and 'discovering' value. Neither word, however, is quite accurate enough. Scheler quotes Carl Jaspers in this regard: 'In love we do not discover values, we discover that everything is more valuable.' In other words, love achieves the enhancement of values already inherent in that which is the object of love.

Scheler makes it clear that love may be of different kinds, not all of them directly relevant to morality – love of beauty for instance or love of country. Moreover, love has its counterpart in hatred, which (like love) is much more than an emotional reaction. It is a consistent action of *dis*valuing that towards which it is directed. Thus a morality based on love must be carefully delineated to show its power to oppose hatred. Sympathy points the way. Moral goodness consists in the love of all our fellow human beings, through empathy, identification, but especially by bringing forth the values they themselves possess. Where hatred constantly seeks to disvalue our fellow humans, love constantly seeks to enhance their value. But here too a paradox appears. The value to be enhanced is the value of other people *in all their inner secrecy.* (Fundamental to Scheler's understanding is the belief that the real world is always much richer than what is given to our immediate awareness. *My* view of other people is a pale representation of what they are in themselves.) So love of persons can proceed only so far as they disclose themselves. Love is creative, but in an enabling, not in a dominating fashion. It is not to be confused with a romantic envelopment of the other which denies separateness and privacy. Scheler quotes Rabindranath Tagore on this point:

> Force me from the bonds of your sweetness, my love!
> . . .
> I am lost in you, wrapped in the folds of your caresses.
> Free me from your spells, and give me back the manhood
> to offer you my freed heart.[18]

He might equally have quoted these lines from Kahlil Gibran's *The Prophet*:-

> Give your hearts, but not into each other's keeping . . .
> And stand together yet not too near together:
> For the pillars of the temple stand apart,
> And the oak tree and the cypress grow not in each other's
> shadow.[19]

2. THE QUESTION OF PURITY

After this excursion into the theoretical background to altruism we may return to the issue of professions and purity. 'Pure and holy will I keep my Life and my Art' states the medical oath attributed to Hippocrates. The words imply an ethos of dedication of a religious kind; and, indeed, Ludwig Edelstein has argued that the Oath originates from the austere doctrines of Pythagorean philosophy, which demanded a strict control of desire in a life of holiness. (This would explain why the Oath has had such an appeal down the centuries of the Christian era.)[20] A similarly austere ethos underlies the Nightingale Pledge. The young ladies of good character, who were encouraged to enter nursing by Miss Nightingale and her followers, were subjected to a strict regime in the enclosed setting of the Nurses' Home. They had perhaps little opportunity to do other than 'pass their lives in purity'![21]

The atmosphere of the present age is opposed to such moralism, and yet the ethical codes of the professions (for example, the ethical code of the American National Association of Social Workers quoted at the beginning of this chapter) continue to use concepts like 'integrity', 'commitment', and 'dedication'. A secular age cannot easily dispense with some kind of professional ethos, it seems. Although holiness is no longer demanded and the private lives of professionals have become a matter of individual, rather than group, morality, the demand for purity remains, seen now in terms of motives for entering the profession and in terms of the quality of the relationships offered to patients or clients.

What then do we make of these claims? Ehrenreich and English, in a book on women healers and the medical profession, describe professionalism as 'élitist and exclusive, sexist, racist and classist'.[22] In previous chapters we noted the cooler (but no less critical) observations of Freidson and others, which describe professionalism as a bid for privilege and power. Is there any force in the commitment to altruism which seems to deny such accusations? An answer may be found by seeing how professional 'love' could now be described, using the ideas of Fromm, Tillich and, especially, Scheler. Tillich's four forms of love will be used to structure the discussion at this point.

Epithymia and eros in professionalism

We should notice first that the purity advocated in the medical and nursing oaths has a clear sexual reference. The oath of Hippocrates warns against seduction of male or female (a warning reiterated in another ancient source, the Hymn of Serapion). The concern with sexuality in the emergent nursing profession in Britain this century is evidenced not only by the extraordinary restrictions on the trainee nurses already mentioned, but by the barring of men from the College of Nursing and from the General Register.[23] Until quite recently the nursing profession (in Britain at least) has been virtually a sisterhood of single women. Male nurses and the older married women and widows who had staffed hospitals and asylums or had nursed in private homes in previous eras did not fit the new professional image.[24]

Sexuality is of concern in medicine and nursing because the doctor and nurse have privileged access to the patient's body in order to offer care or cure. If this privilege is exploited sexually then the whole basis of the professional relationship is eroded.

Certainly the Nightingale and Pythagorean approaches to this problem may be unnecessarily puritanical (perhaps even damaging to a good relationship), but some way of acknowledging the dangerous intimacy of the relationship seems to be required. The *epithymia* (desire) and *eros* (response to the other's body) which also gives vitality to the relationship need channeling by a professional ideal. In a less dramatic, but no less important way, the intrusion of the social worker into people's private lives also needs a commitment to genuine concern to save it from prurience and malicious gossip. The professional social worker is committed to a degree of sensitivity and discretion not necessarily found in the helpful neighbour.

Apart from sexual and quasi-sexual (prurient) desire, one may see other forms of potentially disruptive *epithymia* in professional work. Critics have focused on desires for money and status. Clearly these enter into aspects of professional practice, especially in medicine, where the rewards are higher than in other fields. Yet here we should pay attention to Fromm's observations. The use of other people's distress merely to maximize one's own income would (in his view) evidence a *lack* of self-love. The professional who treats patients without care or respect lacks care and respect also for himself or herself. Fromm would assume that the desire to be helpful to others is a genuine and powerful motivator. This desire would be frustrated by the selfish pursuit of gain. Thus the professional's egoism and altruism are not necessarily antagonistic.

An aspect of *epithymia* and *eros* which we have already noticed in relation to medical practice is the excitement associated with the acquisition of knowledge and skill. George Orwell has a graphic description of this in his essay, 'How the Poor Die':

> . . . if you had some disease with which the students wanted to familiarize themselves you got plenty of attention of a kind . . . It is strange to relate, but sometimes as some young student stepped forward to take his turn at manipulating you he would be actually tremulous with excitement, like a boy who has at last got his hands on some expensive piece of machinery.[25]

Undoubtedly one of the attractions of professional work with the ill and disadvantaged is this sense of participation in a special knowledge of which the lay world knows little or nothing. The pursuit of knowledge is *erotic*, in the sense that it is the pursuit of something valued by the learner. The patient becomes a means to the satisfaction of this *eros*, with no value independent of his or her contribution to the greater accumulation of knowledge. Once again, we see why a professional ethos stressing altruism develops. The skill and knowledge of the health and welfare professions is mostly gained from actual practice, where people's lives and happiness are at risk. The *eros* which aims at knowledge must be controlled by an ethic which stresses the benefit of patients as the first consideration.

Philia and agape in professionalism

As we add the more personal elements of professional care we see a fresh set of complexities. It is a cliché of professional ethics that patients and clients should be treated as 'persons'. Scheler has ably demonstrated how subtly 'fellow-feeling' enters into relationships where such love may act. The notion of fellow-feeling is an attractive one, but it also creates problems for professional relationships. There are contradictory demands upon the professional helper. We might say that a *critical distance* is required between the helper and the person helped – too great a distance prevents the helper from responding to the other's need: too little distance disables the helper from seeing the problem objectively and offering support from outside the situation.

Here we may gain some clarification from Scheler's meticulous categorizing of different types of fellow-feeling: empathy, identification, mutual feeling, vicarious feeling, emotional infection. The professional who cannot participate in the other's feelings (*einfühling* – empathy) is too distant to help: but where *einsfühling* (loss of self in 'identification') occurs there is too much closeness for professional help. We need to distinguish between a professional relationship and a personal friendship (*philia*). With a friend or a relative I may have such a close identification that we resonate to one another's feeling, we feel mutually in certain situations. But it is unreasonable (and in fact unhelpful) to expect professional helpers to have friendships of this quality with those whom they help. They may feel vicariously (as we might feel for a drowning man, as Scheler puts it), but for their own protection and the protection of their patients or clients they must not be taken over by the other's emotion. To develop Scheler's analogy, they must stand at the water's edge ready to throw a rope (or perhaps dive in) but they must not allow themselves to become infected by the drowning man's terror.

It is in the *control* of sympathy that the importance of a professional ethos may again be seen. There is a certain discipline in professionalism acquired through training and experience. Natural reactions to human distress are modified to a point where the professional may seem cold and unfeeling – mutilated and dead bodies are handled with clinical detachment; situations of squalor and degradation are entered without expressions of judgement and disgust; violent emotions are responded to calmly and with understanding. The ideal professional has learned, in Scheler's phrase, 'to elevate himself heroically above his body'. He or she learns to 'allow his instinctive life to look after itself' after years of experience in the clinic, the ward or the social service department.

But the danger of such professionalization is also easily seen. A 'case-centred' approach may be learned which effectively insulates the doctor, nurse or social worker from the individuality of the people seeking their aid. Moreover, the professional often neglects the emotional distress in himself or herself caused by exposure to suffering. The very empathy which might allow this has itself become a technique skilfully adapted to meet different types of cases. The uniqueness of both the self and the other is lost. Thus the greatest problem for the professional helper is the demand for *agape* – the love which risks self in order to enhance value. We recall Scheler's quotation from Jaspers: 'In love we do not discover values, we discover that everything is more valuable.' Tillich's description of the privacy of every centred individual's being is also important here, and so is Scheler's warning against trying to envelop the other with a possessive love. *Agape* requires that no help, however well-intentioned, should stamp out one's own or another's individuality. Genuine help must see each person, including the helper, afresh, as a new and separate being, for whom no real parallel exists in prior experience – the unique encountering the unique.

The requirements of *agape* are, I believe, at the root of the atmosphere of purity and dedication which permeates professional ethics. We must recognize that its requirements are more than can be reasonably expected. I have already criticized Erich Fromm for failing to see the difficulty in combining love of self with love of others. This difficulty is well illustrated by the contradictions of professionalism. The professional gains knowledge in order to help, but that knowledge gives both detachment and power. It is a hard demand that the detachment should not be used for the protection of self, nor the power for the enhancement of self. It is not easy to follow the ideal which Wilkes describes for social work, but which may apply equally to the other professions: the turning of the 'servant' into the 'master' through the use of expertise.[26] Too easily it is the professional who remains master. Thus I would see altruism, in all its complexity now laid out, as entirely appropriate to, indeed necessary for, professional helping. Yet I concede that it is elusive, perhaps possible only as a commitment which is frequently not honoured.

Does this mean, then, that I dismiss out of hand the interpretation of professionalism as the egoistic accumulation of power and privilege? Not so. Undoubtedly professionalism serves these functions also, as even a cursory glance at the rise of professions in modern society will show. Occupational groups may claim that they band together in professional associations solely for the benefit of clients, but they themselves may not be the best judges of that. The fact is that the achievement of professional status brings considerable advantages. We must certainly guard against a false piety about professions and their high ideals. For example, the following quotation from Abraham Flexner about professionalism in social work, while right in stressing altruism, seems unduly idealistic in tone:

What matters most is professional spirit . . . In so far as accepted professions are prosecuted at a mercenary or selfish level, law and medicine are no better than trades . . . The unselfish devotion of those who have chosen to give themselves to making the world a fitter place to live in can fill social work with the professional spirit . . .[27]

But the professions *are* trades. They are ways of making money through the exercise of special knowledge and skills. What sets them apart from other occupations is that they deal with people at times when they are especially vulnerable and unable to help themselves. It is this which requires the addition of love to the quest for mercenary gain.

Thus the socially competitive elements in professionalism should not be denied, but it is not correct to see them as the only elements of importance. Alongside them we may see an appropriate role for professionals as 'moderators of love'. By way of conclusion to this chapter I shall explain in a little more detail what I intend by this phrase.

3. MODERATORS OF LOVE

In speaking of 'moderators of love' I have in mind both ecclesiastical and meteorological nuances of meaning. I refer to an office in Presbyterian polity and to a much prized feature of the climate of temperate zones.

In Presbyterian church government the Moderator keeps order in the Assembly, but possesses no status in himself. He is merely *primus inter pares* (first among equals) and his office is limited in duration (normally one year) to prevent an accumulation of personal power and prestige. The professions are (or should be) moderators of love in this first sense. Since they claim an ethic of *agape*, they stand between the weak and the strong in society. They can ensure that through their work the disadvantages of weakness are evened out and each person is given equal consideration as an individual of worth. They can also draw the attention of those in political office to the injustices which their work uncovers. Thus they have an important social role as mediators. This is especially evident in the community aspects of social work and in what I have called the prophetic role of medicine. But at the same time the power and influence of the professions must be carefully limited. The critique of professionalism by Freidson and others is accurate, to the extent that it uncovers inappropriate and unjustified use of professional influence, both over individual patients and over the society as a whole. Although the professional (unlike the Moderator) does not demit office after a year, there should be no *permanent* status for any profession in relation either to individual patients or to governments.

In the meteorological sense, too, the caring professions can offer 'moderated love'. Here, indeed, their particular skill and social usefulness is most clearly seen. As we have seen, the professional does not and cannot love (or hate) a person as a relative or friend does. There is a necessary detachment in professional care. Yet it *is* love which the professional offers, however moderated. It is a reaching out to another in the desire to enhance the value which is seen, and such reaching-out requires the non-rational connection which feeling alone can create. We employ the professional helper to maintain this balance of reason and emotion. There is a protection for the patient or client in knowing that the professional has a living to earn and a reputation to maintain. There should be a hard-headedness and consistency in the care offered, unlike the more erratic and turbulent attempts to help which emanate from family and friends. In the ideal at least, the climate of professional help is always a moderate one, temperate and without extremes and sudden changes.

Finally, like the Presbyterian Moderator, professional helpers represent more than human attempts to care. Their opposition to illness, pain, and social disadvantage symbolizes the 'impossible ideal'[28] of *agape*, a love which restores full value to every individual, however damaged, however oppressed, however bereft of hope. In this sense the professional commitment is a religious one, though this need not imply that the practitioners see themselves as believers. Their *actions* and *attitudes* look for an ultimate conquest of suffering. Perhaps unrealistically, perhaps arrogantly, they oppose misery, fallibility and death itself. Their commitment expresses a hope which Christians symbolize by speaking of incarnation, crucifixion, resurrection and a final victory when all is made new. The hope which *agape* embodies is total.

Edwin Muir, in a poem which is startling in its theological

novelty, speaks of a final 'transfiguration' which will undo *all* suffering:

> Then he will come, Christ the uncrucified,
> Christ the discrucified, his death undone,
> His agony unmade, his cross dismantled –
> Glad to be so – and the tormented wood
> Will cure its hurt and grow into a tree
> In a green springing corner of young Eden,
> And Judas damned, take his long journey backward
> From darkness into light and be a child
> Beside his mother's knee, and the betrayal
> Be quite undone and never more be done.[29]

Here is the transcendent element to which all attempts to love seem to point. Certainly many may quarrel with the theology of Muir's poem, and many others may feel that such references to Christian symbolism are quite irrelevant to professional care. Yet if the professional commitment to service is genuine (not merely window-dressing to entice public approval), then in all professional work there is some kind of hope in love's triumph. In the final chapters of this book I shall attempt to describe the theological foundations of such 'moderated' love.

SIX

Knowing What Is Best

A professional is someone who knows better what is good
for his client than the client himself does.

Everett Hughes[1]

> He does not think there is anything the
> matter with him because
>   one of the things that is
>   the matter with him
>   is that he does not think that there
>   is anything
>   the matter with him
> therefore
>   we have to help him realise that
>   the fact that he does not think there is
>   anything
>   the matter with him
>   is one of the things that is
>   the matter with him

R.D. Laing[2]

> I am not yet born : O hear me,
> Let not the man who is beast or who thinks
>   he is God come near me.

Louis MacNeice, 'Prayer before Birth.'[3]

I have come now to a transition, a shift toward the more
explicitly theological in an attempt to establish the background
to the moderated love of professional care. But it would be
disingenuous to suggest that my own theological presuppositions have not entered into the argument until now. I make no
claim to a value-free survey of the three professions in the

previous chapters. Clearly my identification of themes like hope, companionship and incarnate knowledge and my choice of the image of moderator for professional care have not simply 'emerged' from the material available. I have deliberately organized it and interpreted it in ways which followed from the assumption that a purely egoistic account of professionalism was insufficient, albeit highly persuasive within its limits. I have sought language to speak realistically, but without unjustified cynicism, about love. In doing this I have tried to keep in dialogue with those writers who see self-interest as the only irreducible form of human motivation and whose view of society leaves no room for genuine altruism. The ambiguity of professional care demands both types of explanation.

My shift toward more explicit theological statements should not be seen as a denial of this ambiguity. There can be no simple theological 'answers', and it should not be supposed that traditional formulations can do justice to the dilemmas of caring for others. In an early poem Eliot described how he was moved by 'the notion of some infinitely gentle, infinitely suffering thing'.[4] This is also the spirit of Christian theology, with its discovery of love in crucifixion, and it must inform every theological quest. There must always be a sense of vulnerability in trying to write theology. In this cautious spirit, three questions will be discussed in the remainder of this book: how do we know what is best for people?; how can we give and receive care in ways that are not demeaning?; and how can love find political expression? These are the central issues which arise in the moderation of love by professional care-givers.

What is best?

The issue to be tackled in this chapter is the nature of professional knowledge. Does the specialized knowledge of doctors, nurses and social workers equip them to know what will most benefit the people who seek their help? Or are patients or clients the best judges of their own welfare? As the argument proceeds, we shall see that neither the client nor the professional can judge what should be done in isolation. Knowledge of what is best must proceed from the meeting between the helper and the helped and even then it will be incomplete and uncertain. It is relatively easy, of course, to describe professional expertise within certain defined limits. The cardiac surgeon knows how to repair damaged heart valves; the nurse knows how to administer drugs; the social worker knows how to advise on welfare benefits. But the search for 'what is best' for a person in need is always more complex than such simple descriptions of standard helping procedures imply. This is so for two reasons: firstly, because all knowledge possessed by the helping professions must cope with the problem of the *application* of what is known to each individual person; secondly, because the knowledge required to help or advise another is never value-free – it entails judgements about how people can become happier, healthier, or more fully human. These two aspects of uncertainty in professional knowledge will be the subject of the reflections which now follow, reflections based on the themes of incarnation, creation and faith.

1. INCARNATION AND LIMITATION

We may begin our discussion with some ecstatic utterances of Dame Julian of Norwich, as she considers the 'shewings' of Christ's passion which she has received:

> Wouldst thou learn thy Lord's meaning in this thing? Learn it well: Love was His meaning. Who showed it thee? Love. What shewed He thee? Love. Wherefore shewed it He? For love.[5]

Dame Julian takes us to the heart of a Christian understanding of 'knowing what is best', an understanding which links knowledge with love and suffering. When it comes to a knowledge of persons which genuinely seeks to help them, there can be no knowledge without pain. This is arguably what is most distinctive about the Christian gospel. Jesus is portrayed in the Synoptic Passion narratives as learning (and thereby revealing) *painfully* the will of the Father, which is the way of love. Nikos Kazantzakis conveys this graphically in his novel *The Last Temptation*, when for a while (as in a dream sequence) Jesus is seen to be settling into comfortable married life and avoiding Calvary – then the dream shatters and his love takes him on to that end he so dreaded in Gethsemane. The

Christian meaning of love is, as Moltmann so succinctly puts it, 'the crucified God' – not the offering of a victim to appease a distant deity, but a love which identified totally with the most despised and rejected of human beings.

The Cross, then, is the revelation of love as involvement, and such involvement is a kind of knowing of personal reality which can be gained in no other way. Even an omniscient God must share our flesh to know us in love's way. There is no knowledge of persons in that which is invulnerable, impassible, eternally detached from the reality of pain. Only the God who is with us is the God who can save us.

This linking of knowledge, love and suffering in theology has profound implications for the knowledge upon which professional care must be based. We have repeatedly seen the danger that the special knowledge of the professional becomes a form of domination. The social worker may seek to impose 'what is best' upon people either in the service of an uncritical social conformism or in the name of a revolution which, it is believed, only a 'false consciousness' would oppose. The nurse may use skill and 'body-expertise' to infantilize or depersonalize patients. The doctor may use scientific knowledge to create inappropriate dependence and ill-founded faith. Against all those forms of domination we can offer the way of 'knowing what is best' which is based on love. This, as Christian symbolism conveys, is both incarnate and vulnerable. It implies three essential features in the knowledge of persons: particularity, mutuality and incompleteness.

Particularity

We encounter in attempts to develop a relevant knowledge for helping others the problem of singularity. All attempts to transmit knowledge about illness or social distress depend upon generalizations. The notion of 'disease', for example, relies upon grouping the signs and symptoms in separate patients into classes, tracing connections which transcend individual variation and eventually developing a model of the disease which allows for reasonably accurate diagnosis and prognosis and reasonably effective curative interventions (if such exist). One might summarize this approach by saying that the disease 'has the patient' rather than that the patient 'has the disease'. The individuality of the patient is important only so far as it complicates the diagnosis or makes the prognosis less certain. We can observe similar generalizations in nursing (for example, the 'senile demented', the 'cardiac case') and in social work (the 'inadequate mother', the 'oppressed minority group'). Admittedly the literature of professional work stresses the importance of returning from such generalizations to the individual case, with all the complexity which that entails, but the *pain* of keeping to knowledge of the particular is rarely sufficiently noticed. It demands the time and attention which professionals can ill afford if they are to respond to all the demands being made upon them. In order to retain a sense of control we need sameness and predictability in our daily experience. We rarely seek out the new and different in *work*, but leave such things to the recreation designed to alleviate the boredom of the predictable, upon which we subsist. But the knowledge, which love seeks, demands the more costly encounter.

In this context, we may see the Christian doctrine of Incarnation in a new light. It has often been maintained that the main scandal of Christianity, its chief absurdity, is that an eternal God is portrayed as being revealed at a specific time, in a particular place and in an individual person. But one can turn this absurdity on its head. Generalization comes easily to the human mind: it is genuine particularity which points to the divine. The discomfort of the unexpected, the wholly new and unpredictable is something we can scarcely tolerate. In comparison, the concept of a timeless omniscience and an unchallenged omnipotence seems easy to contemplate.

At the level of human knowing the considerations of particularity make it inevitable that no person can have adequate knowledge of what is best for the other, if that knowledge is to be regarded as possessed solely by one partner in an interaction. The other must reveal his or her particularity and the true welfare of the other must always be sought by sharing.

Mutuality

Particularity requires mutuality. It is important to notice that this is a mutuality *with the aim of improving knowledge*. William F. May has rightly written some cautionary words against a stress on mutuality which ignores the necessity for skilled knowledge:

> A rather sentimental existentialism unfortunately assumes that it is enough for human beings to be 'present' to one another. But in crisis, the ill person needs not simply presence but skill, not just personal concern but highly disciplined services targeted on specific needs.[6]

Martin Buber, perhaps the main proponent of 'being present', makes the same point in a discussion with the psychotherapist Carl Rogers. Against Rogers' claim that he can offer his patients 'I–thou' relationships, Buber insists that the essential differences between the helper and the helped make such encounters impossible.[7] The patient is inevitably dependent on the helper in a way that the helper is not upon the patient.

Such warnings are necessary to guard against a false egalitarianism that refuses to see the appropriateness of an authority to offer help based on knowledge and experience. Nevertheless, the limits to the knowledge of the helper must also be emphasized. In matters which affect the well-being and the hopes and aspirations of another person the professional helper must rely on the revelation of an inner world of experience, to which there is no access from outside, except so far as the other person chooses to grant it. Max Scheler speaks of the disclosure of the person of another, which can come only by 'joining in the performance of his acts' cognitively and through imaginative identification.[8] The following case from a manual of medical general practice illustrates the point at a relatively trivial, but nonetheless relevant, level:

> Mr J.F., a middle-aged man, came to the surgery to be signed fit for work after an attack of influenza. He said he was still feeling a little run down and would like 'a good old-fashioned tonic.' The doctor, judging him to be of reasonable intelligence and ripe for some health education, suggested to him that a tonic with the usual

ingredients would not benefit him at this juncture. The patient did not receive this very kindly and insisted that he be given a tonic. The doctor, having made his point, felt unable to change his attitude and offer the man a bottle of what he had already described to him as pharmacologically useless liquid. The discussion became quite heated on the patient's part and he departed with a very disgruntled air. He always avoided that partner subsequently.[9]

The doctor had knowledge of the patient's state of health and of the pharmacology of traditional tonics, but he failed to gain knowledge of what the authors of the case study call the patient's 'assumptive world'. He was thus unable to offer help which was acceptable to the patient. This does not mean, of course, that the patient's perception of what will help him is always the best one and that professional knowledge must simply be set aside, if it contradicts what the patient wants. The point is rather that knowledge of what is best is most likely to be gained through a meeting of the *world* of the patient and the *world* of professional knowledge and expertise. Every transaction is an inter-personal one and there is no prior set of solutions for the puzzle of what will be best for a person.

Incompleteness

Perhaps the most painful aspect of such an 'incarnate', vulnerable approach to knowledge is that it is incomplete by its very nature. The quest for certainty in theology illustrates this discomfort well. To have a historically based faith is to be left at the mercy of all the contingency and obscurity of history. Naturally, then, certainty is sought, perhaps in infallible Scripture, or an infallible Church or infallible personal experience. How else can one avoid the terrible relativism of human interpretations (and reinterpretations) of God and his purposes? We feel that somewhere we must find the unchanging and utterly dependable. But the relativity of theological orthodoxy itself is surely a clear enough proof of the hopelessness of this quest. Each age or group may devise final and irrefutable dogma, yet the finality fails to survive and the irrefutability fails to convince even a majority of fellow believers for long. There is forever new business to transact in the theological colloquium!

Thus we may conclude that the unfinished is part of what Christians are given. Christian belief is a point of departure, not a place of arrival, and the journey will sometimes seem fruitless. Of course, Christians look for a final triumph, and base their hope on the resurrection, a guarantee that God has prevailed and will prevail. But the resurrection itself is in history and the hope of final triumph is a prediction about history as yet unseen – the guarantees share in the contingency they are meant to overcome! So Christians are always travellers across the rich and puzzling territory of time. They follow a God who calls, but never compels, whose own commitment to human history gives his followers 'no abiding city'. In such a faith, the search for secure completeness is idolatry.

In this situation, it is best for both professionals and their clients that doctors, nurses and social workers become more honest about how little they can do and how very incomplete the knowledge is upon which they seek to help others. It is always easier to see the mistakes of the past – the demeaning effects of the Poor Law administration, for example, or the damage done to psychiatric patients by medical and nursing practices which we now describe as 'institutionalization'. But we also get many hints of *continuing* mistakes and inadequacies: the over-prescription of drugs, serious failures in child-care policies, ill-treatment of patients in the long-stay wards of subnormality hospitals provide obvious examples.

Such professional honesty is found in the following amusing reminiscences of medical training:

> . . . the hardest lesson I learned at medical school was that health is not to be sought there, and that if perchance it was found, it was not a matter for my attention. None but the sick were to be studied . . . and I was never allowed to diagnose someone as being healthy, but was limited to the traditional cautious statement that he showed no apparent disease.[10]

This is a good warning against a too narrow 'disease-eradication' approach to medicine. At the same time, such a cautious attitude can help remind people that a professional's knowledge of what constitutes *goodness* is really no better than anyone else's.

2. CREATION AND CONNECTEDNESS

To this point the doctrine of incarnation has appeared to be largely negative in effect, limiting human pride by a reminder of fallibility and finitude. But this negativity is balanced by a notably positive element in Christian theology, which may be loosely described as 'Christian humanism'. It is not just that we are beings of particularity and incompleteness. God *affirms* us in our particularity and he promises that our incompleteness has a purpose. The incarnation celebrates the goodness of humanity and it encourages us to seek hope in being the creatures we are. (In theological terms, the doctrine of incarnation leads us back to the doctrine of creation and encourages us to find the future glory which sin has obscured.) The positive features which emerge from this hope in created human nature may be seen to be three forms of connectedness – to one's own body, to other persons and to the physical universe.

Firstly, to be a creature is to be linked to a body in such a total way that all descriptions of the self apart from the body are mere abstraction. Each of us is an 'embodied self', and what is good for us has always a bodily manifestation. Thus, helping a person must entail seeking that which keeps a unity between the self and the body. It is essential to notice the variations between individual people in this regard. A doctrine of creation encourages the metaphor: 'What is *this* body saying?' In a sense, the body's voice *is* the Creator's voice, reminding the person of what could bring an end to the internal strife. The voice may ask for greater relaxation, or greater effort; it may rally forces of self-preservation, or it may cry out to be allowed to age and die. The professional (here especially the doctor and the nurse) uses knowledge and skill to 'tune in' to that voice. At the same time, we must remember that the phrase 'the voice of the body' is *only* a metaphor. We cannot know what is best by ignoring the body, but we need not take the bodily as normative either. The conscious self has a remarkable potential for controlling and altering the body. In order to pay proper attention to this aspect of createdness we must speak of both 'psychosomatic' and 'somatopsychic' influences. The professional helper can be ally of either body or psyche in helping a person restore a lost balance.

Secondly, as creatures we are intimately linked to others. Although we may feel intensely individual and at times acutely alone, we are social beings from the moment of conception to the moment of death. To be a creature is to be born of others, to know ourselves through them, to depend upon them and create dependency, to know the pain of losing them and finally to be the instance of that pain to others. The effort to know what is best for people is thus bound to fail if it is too narrowly individualistic. I referred earlier to the concept of the 'assumptive worlds' of the helper and the helped. These worlds are made up of a network of relationships, whose influences often go unnoticed. The doctor, nurse or social worker is never a wholly autonomous individual, deciding in pure isolation how to offer help. The prior assumptions of upbringing and social class, of professional ethos and of agency policy, all strongly influence how help is offered. Similarly, help is sought out, and accepted or rejected, by patients and clients within the framework of their social environment, which is exceedingly complex, varied and powerful.

How then do we know what is best for people as social beings? Two errors must be avoided. The first sees health and well-being as 'adjustment to society'. What this phrase usually means is conformity to the *helper's* conception of good social relationships. The other extreme is found in an over-emphasis on 'client self-determination' where this implies that the client's assumptive world is beyond criticism. Instead, we need to see that social relationships, from the earliest period of childhood onward, serve two quite different ends – support and growth.[11] A 'good relationship', whether in the family, the neighbourhood, or in the wider context of state-provided services, gives both security and challenge. Both are necessary for our creaturely existence. We need security to survive; we need challenge to live at a level beyond mere survival. The professional, who learns to question his or her own assumptive world, will be in a better position both to give the expected comfort and to help the client grow beyond the assumptions on which help is sought and offered.

Thirdly, as creatures we are connected to the natural world as a whole. (As the Preacher puts it: 'From dust we are made and to dust we shall return.' – Eccles. 12.7) Human beings seem particularly unsure of this aspect of their creatureliness. The desire to possess and dominate the world casts a deep shadow over the created unity of humankind and the natural environment. Indeed so deep is the shadow that even to describe such unity sounds like sheer romanticism. The world is more usually seen as a place of danger or a place for material gain: rarely simply as 'our place'. As creatures we are as linked to the physical universe as we are to our own bodies. There is no other place for us, in life as we know it, and we are in unceasing physical interaction with the physical world which we so distrust and ignore. Yet we draw a boundary at the fringes of our body, disregarding its total dependence on all that surrounds it.

Perhaps, then, it is increasingly on this aspect of creatureliness that the professional who seeks to 'know what is best' must concentrate. Medicine is slowly gaining an awareness of the environmental dimensions of human health and ill-health. The awareness begins with the identification of noxious environmental influences created by industrialization, but it is beginning to expand to include a broader understanding of the 'diseases of civilization', which have resulted from the changed relationships between human beings and the natural world as a whole. This new thinking encompasses methods of agriculture and associated dietary habits, styles of work, the use of the environment in recreation, architecture and town-planning, modes of transport, design of furniture, of clothing and of working implements. A similar expansion of awareness is required in nursing and social work, in relation to noxious institutional and community environments, and more widely to the recuperative effects of contact with living and growing things.[12]

Of course, an emphasis on this aspect of creatureliness must avoid the myth of the 'noble savage'. Primitive styles of living are neither particularly healthy nor necessarily productive of human fulfilment. The environment we inhabit is one which has been modified to great advantage by human ingenuity. A 'return to nature' could mean merely a return to a brief and uninspiring life of physical toil. The point is rather that we must not allow ourselves to be so impressed by our techno-logical adaptiveness that we fail to see how much it destroys in the name of progress. There are rhythms, harmonies and balances in nature to which we seem to respond with a sense of joyful recognition. These too reflect the goodness of creation, just as bodily existence and human relationships do. To disregard such basic aspects of our creaturely existence results in the helpers and the helped seeing only diseases, disorders and problems, never a vision of what is best for humankind. To know what is best is to help oneself and the other recover the lost richness of the world we so briefly inhabit.

3. FAITH AND FOOLISHNESS

Finally, however, even the positive aspects to be found in an understanding of the connectedness of creation fail to satisfy. Earlier we noted the restless, adventuresome character of human life, which, as Dubos and Wilson observe, has to be included in any equation about health and well-being (see chapter 2). In the theological terminology I am now employing, we need to add to incarnation and creation the hope of resurrection.

Daniel Day Williams describes love as 'that experience of spirit which has communion in freedom as its goal'.[13] The definition reminds us of other definitions of its kind, for example, Scheler's account of the active valuing of love or Tillich's of love as the power of being. If we are going to describe professional care as in service of such love, then we must set our sights higher than the doctrine of creation will allow. The best for us, as Christian belief understands it, is not a return to Eden. It is more than a making peace between self and body, self and others, self and world, however necessary and important such a restored harmony may be. The foolishness of faith seeks a new kind of reconciliation in which the glory of God shines fully in all the created order, and human freedom leads, not to self-absorption and destructive-ness, but to creativity and a joyous sharing.

This foolishness (for, by the world's standards such ideas are the mere illusions of religion described by Freud) is promoted by a different kind of knowing. Worship, sacrament and private prayer all sustain Christians in such foolish hopes. Here sacrament holds a special place, since it uses the material substances of water, bread and wine as a focus for transformations which reach beyond intellectual understanding. Distinctions between matter and spirit break down in such celebrations of sacramental hope, just as in private prayer time's barriers are broken and in public worship the restrictions of space fall away. Holy things, holy times and holy places are simply the ordinary items of our world illuminated by a different kind of knowing. George Herbert has a remarkable poem about prayer which conveys this well:

> A kind of tune, which all things hear and fear;
> Softness, and peace, and joy, and love, and bliss,
> Exalted manna, gladness of the best,
> Heaven in ordinary, man well drest,
> The milky way, the bird of Paradise,
> Church-bells, beyond the stars heard, the soul's blood,
> The land of spices; something understood.[14]

What can such religious sentiments have to do with secular helping professions? The foolishness of faith may seem irrelevant to those who do not share in Christian faith or worship in Christian communities. Yet perhaps one should not too readily assume this. There may be a sacramental dimension to helping outside the context of explicit Christian commitment. (Robert Lambourne has described this dimension as the 'sacrament of the cup of cold water'.[15]) Many examples could be given: the element of faith which leads to the 'placebo effect' in medical treatment; the measured ritual of clinic and hospital which transcends their utilitarian function; the nurse's ministrations to the body, living or dead, which can communicate a respect beyond the requirements of health or hygiene; the body language of the social worker which communicates to people a physical presence beyond bureaucratic necessity. We enter here a territory which is very difficult to talk about without a descent into vague sentimentality. Nevertheless, the effort to heal, to care for, or to support emotionally, resists specification in precise tasks for which knowledge at an intellectual level is appropriate. There is something beyond this which makes professional work an effort to express the foolishness of faith in the temples and rituals of a secular religion.[16]

Knowing Sacramentally

I have been suggesting throughout this chapter that 'knowing what is best' is a complex and elusive notion. A central difficulty may be found in the particularity of people's problems and the inevitable incompleteness and relativity of human knowledge. Certainly some hints toward a theology of health, which could give guidance for professional interventions, have been found in the connectedness of our creaturely existence. Eventually, however, what is good for us is so bound up with the restlessness of the human spirit that our minds cannot encompass what is required. We are led to the non-rational in professional work, where help is given in mysterious ways. This domain of the 'sacrament of the cup of cold water' will be charted in the next chapter, as we explore the subtleties of caring and being cared for.

SEVEN

Caring and Being Cared For

Just as the person who comes to me needs me for help, I
need him to express my ability to give help.

James Hillman[1]

The first enters wearing the neon armour
Of virtue
Ceaselessly firing all-purpose smiles
At everyone present
She destroys hope
In the breasts of the sick
Who realize instantly
That they are incapable of surmounting
Her ferocious goodwill

Charles Causley, 'Ten Types of Hospital Visitor'[2]

Love means willingness to participate
in the being of the other at the cost
of suffering, and with the expectation of
mutual enrichment, criticism and growth.

D. Day Williams[3]

The conclusion of the previous chapter brought us to the point
where the relationship between the helper and the helped was
seen to have a transcendent aspect, suggesting not just
knowledge but also the 'foolishness of faith', leading to a
sacramental understanding of caring. By 'sacrament' we may
understand an outward and physical sign, usually conveyed in
bodily action (washing, feeding, anointing, touching), of a
reality which eludes rational description. Now we must look
more closely at this idea. Is it possible to see a theological
dimension in caring, one which is other than the 'rhetoric of

self-advancement' with which professions often surround themselves?

In exploring this question I shall consider first the advantages and disadvantages of describing a professional relationship in terms of 'covenant' rather than of 'contract'. I shall identify two features of the conventional relationship which appear to give it a special character: faithfulness and spontaneity. Despite these special features, however, covenants (like contracts) also have a necessary element of exchange. I shall therefore explore the mutuality (or reciprocity) of the covenantal relationship, which needs emphasizing to avoid the dangers of paternalism and over-zealous helping. This will take us from the idea of covenant to the idea of grace, especially as this expresses itself in bodily forms of caring.

1. CONTRACT AND COVENANT

In his writings on medical ethics, the moral theologian, Paul Ramsey, expresses powerfully the idea that the professional relationship is to be viewed in terms of the biblical concept of covenant. In the Preface to the *Patient as Person* he writes:

> We are born within covenants of life with life. By nature, choice, or need we live with our fellow men in roles or relations. Therefore we must ask, What is the meaning of the *faithfulness* of one human being to another in every one of these relations?[4]

Ramsey goes on to state that in discussing medical ethics he will 'not be embarrassed to use as an interpretative principle the biblical norm of fidelity to covenant'.[5] We should notice, however, that Ramsey's move from the social nature of human beings to his 'interpretative principle' of fidelity to covenant is by no means the simple step he seems to imply. He appears to be canvassing presuppositions about fidelity, without showing why these are especially appropriate to professional helping relationships. If we are to speak of covenants in professional relationships, then we must explain why contracts are not enough, why fidelity is essential. This issue is explored with some care by William F. May in a paper entitled, 'Code, Covenant, Contract or Philanthropy'.[6] The discussion which follows is based largely on May's exposition.

We should note first that there are considerable *similarities* between contracts and covenants. Both entail an agreement between parties which imposes mutual obligations. The biblical covenants might be summed up in the formula: 'If you obey me, you will be my chosen people' (Exod. 19.5), and in the Old Testament we find God continually lamenting his people's broken promises. May describes covenant and contract as 'first cousins', but he goes on to argue that although they have material similarities, they differ radically *in spirit*. Contracts define a precise set of relationships, and, if these are correctly observed, then the contractual obligation is fully discharged. But covenants 'have a gratuitous, growing edge to them that nourishes rather than limits relationships'.[7] We see this in the development of the idea of covenant in the Old Testament: God's steadfast love constantly attempts to win back his people (Jer. 30); despite Israel's unfaithfulness, her lover still seeks her out (Hosea 2.19–23); God is angry at being betrayed, but his anger will not endure for ever (Hosea 11.8–9). Moreover, while contracts imply no more than a *quid pro quo*, covenants contain an element of promise which resists precise specification. The calculation of whether both parties have equal opportunity for gain is alien to the spirit of covenants, but it is central to the concept of a just contract. There is also a communal aspect to covenants. Whereas contracts are typically between two parties, each of whom is regarded as an individual with certain rights to be safeguarded, covenants often define communal relations, a set of interlocking obligations binding a whole group or nation in a common cause. Finally, covenants begin with a gratuitous act, a gift, and this element of spontaneous giving characterizes the continuing relationship.

It might appear that covenant is the more adequate concept for describing the relationship between client and professional helper, but we must avoid too hasty a conclusion on this point. The notion of contract, with its emphasis on mutual advantage, equal obligation and clearly specified criteria for breach of the agreement, has much to commend it. A contractual approach can protect the clients of professionals against paternalism and exploitation. If the obligations of doctors, nurses and social workers are left ill-defined, then it is very difficult for people to know whether they have grounds for complaint. The air of mystery which surrounds professional work can be used to conceal serious error, inadequate standards of work and outright fraud. Moreover, the notion of exchange serves to remind the people who consult professionals that they too have obligations and that they cannot expect continuing help if they refuse to respect the helper's judgement or if they make unreasonable demands.

On the other hand, the contractual relationship appears to give insufficient weight to certain features of professional care. Firstly, those who need the help of a doctor, nurse or social worker are rarely in the position of buyers on the open market, who can protect their interests on the principle, *caveat emptor* ('Let the buyer beware'). Illness and worry impair people's judgement and may encourage them to make hasty and ill-considered attempts to gain help. They must rely on offers of help which are genuinely concerned for their welfare, not merely attempts to gain maximum financial or other advantage for the 'seller' of help. Secondly, the person seeking help is rarely sufficiently well informed about the problem to be able to specify precisely what is expected from the 'seller' of services. A 'contract' can be defined in only the vaguest of terms and the client must rely largely on professional expertise to specify precisely what should be done to help. Thirdly, a contractual approach may encourage both 'minimalism' and 'defensive over-treatment' by professionals. In minimalism the client is given only as much as is economically worthwhile for the professional to offer. In defensive over-treatment professionals protect their own interests by an excess of treatment in order to safeguard themselves against lawsuits. In neither case is the interest of the client paramount.

We may conclude that by encouraging a view of helping relationships as covenants rather than contracts we may avoid the calculation of the more and the less, based solely on self-interest, which leads to the neglect of the true welfare of clients. The professional has a commitment to people, which is not limitless certainly, but which promises more active concern and open-ended helpfulness than the restrictive language of contract implies. Ramsey may, therefore, be correct in describing the professional helping relationship as one of 'covenantal fidelity.'

2. RECIPROCITY

The Need to be Needed

There are, however, considerable dangers in too fervent a support for the concept of fidelity, if this is taken to imply a kind of saintlike condescension by the professional, a heroic dedication to the needy with no thought of reward. We have already observed that contract and covenant are 'first cousins' and, although there is an element of gratuitousness in covenant, there is also reciprocity. Both parties to a covenant are recipients of gifts; neither is just a selfless giver. It is not simply that the professional helper makes a living out of being helpful to others, though this should never be overlooked. There are also more subtle rewards. The choice of a career of caring for people in need presumably stems from some needs in the helper, which gain satisfaction when one's working life is spent in an encounter with illness or social disability. The needy person obviously needs to be helped: but that help most likely comes from someone who needs to be needed. Unless we recognize the element of personal need leading people into professional caring, we shall fail to see how damaging some forms of over-commitment can be. One thinks of the 'ferocious goodwill' of Charles Causley's first type of hospital visitor, which 'destroys hope in the breasts of the sick'. The detachment or emotional neutrality of professionals is meant to protect people against such dangerous dedication. As William May puts it: 'It will not do to pretend to be the second person of the Trinity, prepared to make with every patient the sympathetic descent into his suffering . . . It is important to remain emotionally free so as to be able to withdraw the self when [one's] services are no longer pertinent.'[8]

James Hillman has described in *Insearch* the influence of archetypal symbols of healing and salvation on modern helpers' conceptions of their task. Ancient symbols, suggests Hillman, are often combined with early experiences in which the theme of rescue is prominent, for example, the helpless child who must be saved from a wicked parent.[9] Such unconscious motivations inflate the importance of the help offered to cosmic dimensions, and make a constant supply of needy people a psychic necessity. The *need* to be helpful becomes an insistent *demand* to be perpetually rescuing people. In an article entitled 'The Helping Personality' Hugh Eadie has made some similar observations, based on his research into the health of Scottish clergy. He describes people so anxious to be loving that they continually feel guilty at falling short of the impossible ideal that they have set themselves.[10]

The picture we get from such writings suggests, rather paradoxically, that the truly needy person in some helping relationships may well be the helper. Sick and disadvantaged people are sought out to fill an inner loneliness. Here is how the poet Paris Leary portrays such a person, a priest whose good works bring him admiration and gratitude, but no assuagement of his own needs:

> 'He's frightfully good at coping', Andrew said,
> 'though arthritis makes him snap a bit.
> But he's got all the gen on rules of life,
> and everyone at Bart's, of course, adores him.
> The clergy house is a sort of Coventry-
> cum-hospital . . .
>   He's frightfully good
> at coping, you know. They all end up here.' . . .
> Stiff in the chair which grows and grows around him
> he sits as the dull shilling burns away.
> 'Andrew', he whispers. He cries, 'Andrew', crying
> for young Andrew and the dozens, dozens . . .[11]

Gratitude

The disturbing element in such need-driven caring is that it undermines the spontaneity and gratuitousness which characterizes a covenant relationship. The over-committed helper appears to eschew all personal comfort and private interest in the name of service to others. The reality, however, is often quite other. The hidden rewards are so great that this seeming selflessness is a form of self-assertion, which seeks to deny the reciprocity in all acts of caring and to keep the helper firmly in the ranks of the strong and the need-free.

Three inter-related ideas – gift, gratitude and grace – can help to give a different perspective on this issue. We may restore reciprocity to helping relationships if we emphasize gratitude in the *helper* as well as the helped. This gratitude stems from the experience of receiving gifts, which made the giving of care possible. The Christian belief in calling or vocation expresses this in terms of *charisma*, an ability one possesses as a result of God's grace, not through any personal merit. Those who work in the 'caring professions' are the recipients of such *charismata*. They have gifts of intelligence and personality which enable them to practise a profession in a skilled and effective manner. Their work gives them a sense of fulfilment, of putting to use that which they have been given, and thus of expressing themselves in helping others. So professional care becomes a response to gifts, an act of gratitude, which has its own reward, rather than an act of grudging labour seeking some other satisfaction.

Moreover, part of the reward in such work is the personal character of the relationships which it creates. Using gifts for caring is productive of more gifts from those who are cared for. Frequently the patients of doctors and nurses feel a deep sense of gratitude or indebtedness for the help they have received and they want to express this in monetary or material terms. But the professional, who is aware of how much he or she gains in support, enlightenment and personal development from helping others, may well feel a greater indebtedness. It is often more blessed to care than to be cared for; and the ability to care is frequently made possible by the understanding and sensitivity of the needy person. Such reciprocity suffuses the relationship of caring with a spontaneity, with a sense of grace which enriches carer and cared-for alike.

3. THE GRACE OF CARING AND BEING CARED FOR

A closer examination of grace in caring requires an exploration of the relationship between grace and gracefulness. We feel cared for when *our* need is recognized and when the help which is offered does not overwhelm us but gently restores our strength at a pace which allows us to feel part of the movement to recovery. Conversely, a care which imposes itself on us, forcing a conformity to someone else's ideas of what we need, merely makes us feel more helpless and vulnerable. The experience of being cared for, rather than being 'managed', is summed up in the adjective 'graceful'. Graceful care refers to something which is not offered by anxious people trying to earn love, but by sensitive people who release us from bonds of our own making in spontaneous and often surprising ways. The gracefulness in caring is as closely connected to bodily expression as it is to an intellectual understanding or emotional awareness. The body gracefully offers and gracefully receives, in harmony with thought and feeling. Here especially spontaneity (or lack of it) is seen.

By way of illustration of this theme we may consider two quite unusual stories from the New Testament accounts of the ministry of Jesus, each concerned with an overtly physical form of caring – the anointing of the body with oil or ointment. A notable feature of both stories is that they portray women ministering to Jesus, against voices of protest from the male company who witness the events.

Anointing by a 'sinful' woman

The first story (Luke 7.36–50) describes how a woman 'who lived a sinful life' washed Jesus' feet with her tears, dried them with her hair, kissed them and anointed them with perfume. The sensuous detail in the story may well underline the sense of freedom she feels from the exploitation of her own body in the past. Stressing the idea of gratitude in the woman's actions, Jesus tells the parable of the man who owed little and the man who owed much and concludes, 'whoever has been forgiven little, shows only a little love'. These words of understanding are apparently matched by the physical responses of Jesus. He accepts the woman's tender caresses, despite the disapproval of his host. He gives care by receiving care and he does so in a graceful, bodily way.[12]

The sensuous aspect of such anointing is one which has been given too little attention, because of a tendency to confuse sensuousness with sensuality. Sensuousness is an acceptance and celebration of our senses: sensuality the exploitation of them. Anointing is sensuous, but not necessarily sensual, because it provides comfort and relaxation to a strained or tired body, restoring the person's sense of being 'at home' in the body and renewing mobility and strength. These features may underlie the ancient practice of anointing the sick which is commended elsewhere in the Bible (James 5.14f.), and they are to be seen in the physical care which doctors and nurses provide for bedridden patients. Such acts are genuinely caring when they are gracefully administered, that is to say, carried out in a way which is appropriately sensuous, with a tender respect for the disabled person.

Anointing for burial

The second story (Mark 14.3–9 and parallels) describes the anointing of the head of Jesus by an unnamed woman. The perfume she uses is so costly that some of the onlookers protest at the extravagance. The reply of Jesus makes his awareness of his own need very plain. He does not deny the needs of the poor, but he praises the act because it ministers to him as he approaches an inevitable death. Here is a care which sees *his* need and he is grateful for it. Elisabeth Moltmann-Wendel comments on the implications of this story for an understanding of Jesus' humanity:

> This Jesus needs people. He is not the solitary hero. He is not so sovereign that he can do without his neighbour . . . The luxurious anointing comes from the comforting proximity of women: a delight, enjoyment, pleasure in a solitude that is becoming increasingly painful.[13]

The connection between anointing and death is perhaps as important as its sensuous connotations. The embalming of dead bodies or the use of ointments to delay and conceal putrefaction is an acknowledgement of our fleshly nature. At our death we may receive this last service of others, the gentle and respectful handling of our 'mortal remains'. So in moments of weakness in our lives, the person who cares gracefully for us is like the unnamed woman, acknowledging and helping us to accept our mortality. Much is communicated and shared in the simplest of bodily ministrations.

Sexuality and Gracefulness

We have now seen two examples in which women respond to Jesus' bodily needs. In discussing sexual stereotypes in an earlier chapter (see chapter 3) we saw that while women should not be relegated to merely a subordinate, 'handmaiden', role they do in fact show a greater interest than men in responding to the emotional needs of others. It is perhaps not surprising, then, that in the gospels it is women who are the ministers to Jesus, while the male disciples misunderstand him, fall asleep, or deny him at his time of greatest need. It is the women who offer a costly caring, though the men might equally be capable of it. It is the women whose bodily care gives comfort to Jesus, while the men struggle for places of honour.

Ideally such graceful caring should be accessible to men and women alike. But it is clear that (whether because of nature or nurture) men find it difficult to offer and receive care in a physical way, perhaps fearing that their masculinity will be under threat or that their action or reaction will be interpreted as a sexual advance. The psychoanalyst Ian D. Suttie has written of the 'taboo on tenderness' and he draws attention to the phenomena of male societies or brotherhoods which seem to be attempting to give covert expression to the prohibited feelings of tenderness in men. Suttie believes that there is a primal need to give and receive bodily expressions of tenderness. The caressing of companionship, Suttie argues, is earlier in human development and ultimately more important than sexual arousal. The need to be touched, held and nurtured is with us from the very beginning to the very end of life.[14]

There is something very basic, then, in the experience of being cared for. Each of us knew it in the tender embrace of our mother – that is our first (and perhaps our most important) bodily awareness of grace. All human acts of caring mediate a grace which knows and sustains the person as the mother knows and nurtures the child. Yet these acts must also be appropriate to the situation in which care is required. For the professional person, offering care to a wide variety of people within the context of specific needs, there can rarely (if ever) be the closeness and constancy of a mother's love. This would be inappropriate in most circumstances and would lose sight of the autonomy and coping capacity of the person helped. But although (as I have been suggesting throughout this book) the love of professional care is a *moderated* one, and so should not be confused with the more intimate forms of love we receive from parent or friend, there remains the important element of gracefulness in caring, whose similarity to maternal tenderness and sexual intimacy must not be overlooked. The covenantal relationship, which promotes trust and mutuality, requires bodily mediation in order for its true value to be appropriated by helped and helper alike. The 'sacrament' of caring is the use of the physical closeness of bodies to a therapeutic end, the overcoming of weakness and the restoration of hope which another human presence makes possible.

4. BROTHERLINESS, COMPANIONSHIP AND HOPEFULNESS IN CARING

We are now in a position to look back to the images of caring, which were used in previous chapters to epitomize the relationships of each professional group surveyed, and to see their sacramental character, that is to say, the way in which their physical nature mediates a transcendent love.

We recall that an essential aspect of the medical relationship is the use of knowledge to restore bodily integrity, to welcome back the stranger into the human community and to challenge the health-denying features of contemporary society. This 'brotherly' or 'sisterly' work of medicine is sacramental in character because no physical explanation in terms of disease-eradication or restoration of function can do full justice to its aims. Medical practice deals with living, self-conscious social beings, not merely with isolated parts of organisms. When genuine care is offered to patients (many of whom can have no hope of physical recovery) only the startling imagery of Edwin Muir's 'Christ the recrucified'[15] can portray the message which this care represents. The consistent attention which a humane doctor offers a damaged fellow human being reveals a vision behind the Cross to the young wood in a green corner of Eden. (This can certainly become *hubris*, that vying with God to which medical practice is so prone, and it may lead to a 'heroic' medicine which denies our mortality, but it need not be arrogance of this kind.) A caring response to someone who may soon die creates and discovers the value which cannot be destroyed. It refuses to discard the person because the organism is decaying. This is the secular sacrament of medical care.

In a similar way, the companionship of nursing care provides through physical means a transcendent encouragement which can lead to recovery or to an acceptance of the irremediable. The nurse's actions are, as we have already observed, reminiscent of the mother's care of an infant. The most basic activities of eating, sleeping, excretion and ensuring bodily comfort generally become part of the nurse's concern when a person is seriously ill. In addition, the presence of the nurse is as important to the anxious patient as is the mother's to the frightened child. The nurse often becomes the interpreter to the patient of matters which are perhaps only half understood or half heard when first communicated by the doctor. These features of the nursing relationship make the care which nurses offer their patients an especially powerful means for good or ill. The nurse as companion possesses that gracefulness which we have identified at the heart of caring. There is a sensitivity in companionship which shares without invading privacy and which helps in the other's journey without attempting to dominate and create crippling dependency. When such sensitivity is lacking all the unhelpful features of idealization, demeaning maternalism and stigmatization of unpopular patients which were discussed earlier make nursing care into a health-denying force. But the nurse who offers companionship to patients, even those who seem incapable of much reaction or positive response, embodies the value-creating love, which (to recall Muir's poem once more) helps the tormented wood to cure its hurt. The physical act points to a transcendent reality. The sacramental element is the loyalty of simple care.

Finally, in social work, the gracefulness of caring is found in a stalwart commitment to personal and communal renewal. (Judas a child once more at his mother's knee?) Of the three professions surveyed, social work appears most removed from the physical, most caught in verbalization without concomitant practical action. No doubt this explains the virulence of the debate about the nature of social work and especially about whether radical political change can be one of its objectives. But if we resist the polarization of the personal and the political we may begin to discern the sacramental aspect of social work.

Earlier (in chapter 4) I described the 'dimensions of hope' in the social-work relationship. More than any other profession (except perhaps the clerical profession, which is not under discussion in this volume) social work is obliged to see people 'four-dimensionally'. Precisely because they offer no physical treatment – indeed, rarely any kind of bodily contact – social workers are prevented from relying on one method of helping to the exclusion of the complexities of the client's life and special context. This is evident from the history of social work, which reveals perpetual disenchantment with the favoured method of the previous generation. First the Poor Law and 'welfare worker' image, with its emphasis on handing out material benefits, had to be discarded; then psychoanalytically influenced casework, with its predilection for self-determination and insight, was revealed as masking social injustice; then advocacy for client's rights was challenged as insufficiently radical in its political involvement; now we find questioning about whether politically radical social work can honestly claim to be social work at all, and whether the emerging emphasis on systems theory and change-agency is too managerial and manipulative. Of course, social work is not unique in this tendency to have a succession of fashionable theories, but the range of theory and the rapidity of change is unusual and it reveals the elusive character of social-work action.

How then may a sacramental significance be found in so diverse and ill-defined an activity? An adequate answer to this question must await the final chapter of this book, in which I attempt to describe a theological image of 'the politics of love'. Provisionally, however, we may recall the theme of hope based on four-dimensional perception. The social worker's care is one which enriches the client's self-perception and the perception of the client by others through patient and persistent emphasis on complexity and change. Thus social work care is a sacrament of the future, a set of actions which mediate hope for individuals, families and neighbourhoods simply by refusing to dismiss them as inadequate, beyond remedy, better forgotten. This insistence on hopeful, multi-dimensional perception means that there can be no split between individual and society in social work. Any attempt to insulate the political from the personal merely results in an impoverishment of one's understanding of the person. Social work heralds more forcefully than the other professions, the signs of the times in which an uncaring society brings not only the sad harvest of broken people but also, unless there is change and renewal, its own destruction.

The forms of love

We may note, by way of conclusion, that the transitions through which my discussion of caring have gone mirror to a large extent the different forms of love outlined in my earlier exploration of professional motivation (chapter 5). By rejecting contract in favour of covenant and thereby emphasizing spontaneity, gratitude, faithfulness and gracefulness, I have been tipping the balance away from the predominately self-satisfying motives (*epithymia* and *eros*) toward identification with others (fellow-feeling, *philia*) and toward gratuitous concern for their welfare (value-enhancing love, *agape*). It is important to remember that this is no more than the tipping of a delicate balance slightly to one side. I am not in any sense eliminating self-interest from the 'sacramental' actions of professionals. They are actions of ordinary human beings in which personal need plays an essential part. But they *are* sacramental, when they also mediate a transcendent love which is not confined by egoistic boundaries.

It now remains to describe that wider sweep of *agape* which encompasses social justice. There is a danger that 'brotherliness' and 'companionship' could be short-sighted, even self-indulgent, but the hopeful vision of social work reminds us that we also need a *politics* of love. In the final chapter the paradox of this requirement, that love should seek political ends, will be confronted.

EIGHT

The Politics of Love

She looked over his shoulder
    For vines and olive trees,
Marble well-governed cities
    And ships upon untamed seas.

But there on the shining metal
    His hands had put instead
An artificial wilderness
    And a sky like lead.
        W.H. Auden, 'The Shield of Achilles'[1]

Love seems at best a whisper of the spirit in the clamour
of history.

                                D.D. Williams[2]

Time's handiworks by time are haunted,
And nothing now can separate
The corn and tares compactly grown,
The armorial weed in stillness bound
About the stalk; these are our own.
Evil and good stand thick around
In the fields of charity and sin
Where we shall lead our harvest in.
        Edwin Muir, 'One Foot in Eden'[3]

In the opening chapter of this book I criticized Paul Halmos
for driving a wedge between personal caring and political
change and I argued that one's view of love is inadequate if it
does not encompass questions of social justice. Now I must
substantiate this criticism by attempting to show how
professional 'love' may gain political expression. This is a still

115

more pressing requirement in view of my intervening exposition of the nature of professional care. My descriptions of the moderated love which professionals offer have not been confined to the quality of their relationships with individual clients, important as these are. Many wider questions have arisen. One cannot discuss nursing care without encountering the social issues of sexual stereotyping and the character of the institutions where nurses work. An analysis of medical practice uncovers the political dimensions of socially caused illness and disability and the influence of doctors on health-care policy. Social work, despite its traditional emphasis on the individual client, is enmeshed in political issues, at local, regional and national levels. One may choose to disregard the political dimensions of professional care, but their existence can scarcely be denied.

It may be less obvious, however, that the 'love' which professionals offer has a political dimension. No doubt my phrase 'the politics of love' has an exciting ring to it,[4] but does it have any real meaning? How can politics, the 'art of the possible' which seeks a balance of interests, be an expression of love? It must be admitted that the phrase is an over-confident one if it seems to imply that some kind of transformation of political life can be achieved, whereby competing interests would be set aside in favour of unrewarded altruism or power surrendered in a spontaneous gesture of good will to the disadvantaged. Even if the spirit of St Francis were to possess those in power in this way, one can hardly imagine the saintliness surviving in the political vacuum which would follow! It is idealistic and impractical to imagine that competitiveness can be abolished. The issue rather is whether it can be contained or even reduced by the concern for the good of others which professional care represents. To speak of the politics of love is to consider whether love can be a political influence, bringing about changes in social life, and, if so, how it might operate.

In considering this question I shall refer first to an approach to the philosophy of social welfare described in a phrase coined by Richard Titmuss – the 'gift relationship'. I shall then consider how theological doctrines of sin and salvation modify the optimism of this approach. This will lead on to a discussion of the image of a loving community as a body whose head is Christ, since this theological theme has wider implications than some ecclesiastical interpretations have suggested. Finally, on the basis of this description of 'love's body', I shall return to the question of how professional care may have political influence.

1. THE GIFT RELATIONSHIP

Richard Titmuss' book, *The Gift Relationship*, is ostensibly a study of the voluntary donation of blood, but it soon becomes evident that inherent in this discussion is a basic contribution to social philosophy – a promotion of the concept of 'the freedom to give'. Titmuss describes the relationships exemplified by that between the donors of blood and the potential recipients as 'stranger relationships', because they 'lie outside the reciprocal rights and obligations of family and kinship in modern society'.[5] Although voluntary blood donation is a striking example of such relationships, Titmuss sees it as merely illustrative of what he calls 'creative altruism', which can find expression in the whole philosophy of welfare enshrined in the welfare state. As opposed to market models of health and welfare, the gift relationship describes a different social policy, one which enables people 'to be free to choose to give to unnamed strangers'.[6]

These ideas of Titmuss have been developed by David Watson in his book on the philosophy of social policy, entitled *Caring for Strangers*.[7] Watson agrees with the emphasis on giving in social relationships, drawing a distinction (first formulated by Boulding[8]) between economic policy, which depends on 'bilateral transfer' or exchange, and social policy which depends on 'unilateral transfer', or grants and gifts. The unilateral transfer in social policy is based upon our sense of obligation to 'anonymous others', an obligation which stems not from a motive of gain but from the recognition of our fellow humanity. Thus social policy, in devising structures through which this sense of obligation can be put into practical effect, has an integrative and educative function, creating a more co-operative and caring society. Watson, however, differs from Titmuss in one important aspect. While Titmuss regards gift relationships as 'ultra-obligations', that is, as a giving to others beyond the bounds of duty, Watson believes that there are some 'basic gifts' which we all owe to others. The example of blood donation, from which Titmuss starts, may well be seen as an act of helpfulness to others beyond the strictly morally obligatory: but ensuring that others have their basic rights fulfilled (here Watson has in mind the rights defined in the UN Declaration of Human Rights) is a fundamental moral obligation. So Watson argues that social policy must first devise methods whereby a society grants all its members their basic rights to a minimum standard of living. Then, on this foundation, it should provide opportunities for the 'ultra-obligations' to which Titmuss refers, the overcoming of the spirit of competitiveness through the 'flowering of altruism'.

We may now summarize the 'gift relationship' approach to the politics of love as follows: the best way of ensuring that society 'cares for strangers' is to reduce the atmosphere of competitiveness generated by treating health and welfare as commodities to be bought and sold, and to create structures for the enhancement of giving to others. This may be achieved by the creation of a welfare state, provided the approach to welfare sets everyone free to *give*. A form of welfare which creates a deep division between the professional providers of care and the stigmatized recipients of it does not promote altruism, merely a new form of divisiveness. Professional help should elevate the client's status as a moral agent, setting him or her free to be a *giver*. The norm for the caring society is not the professional helper but the 'ordinary person' who wants to give help to others beyond conventional expectations or legal requirements. Such people are the foundation of a social life which transcends sectional interests and personal gain and which creates new structures for the expression of altruism.

There is considerable power and attractiveness in a theory of this type, but it is nevertheless somewhat vulnerable to the criticism that examples of politically influential 'gift relationships', apart from donations of blood and (possibly) organs for transplantation, are hard to find. In the current climate of economic stringency the concept of the welfare state which has been influential in Britain and in other European countries is steadily being eroded by those who wish the freedom to purchase 'superior' forms of care in a private sector. Thus a social philosophy widely accepted in times of economic buoyancy is quickly set aside when the cost of maintaining it becomes too great for those who can afford to secure their own interests by other means. It seems then that such a view of the politics of love falls under the Marxist critique of 'liberal reformism' – because it fails to confront economic realities, it is easily ignored if it seriously challenges the distribution of wealth and power in a society. Such an approach is indeed in danger of being what D.D. Williams describes as 'a whisper . . . in the clamour of history'.[9]

2. IMPOSSIBLE POSSIBILITIES

A more realistic approach to the politics of love must take account of what Edwin Muir describes in the imagery of the parable of the harvest:

> . . . nothing now can separate
> the corn and tares compactly grown . . .
>
> Evil and good stand thick around
> In the fields of charity and sin
> Where we shall lead our harvest in.[10]

Muir is pointing to the pervasiveness of sin which has every appearance of remaining with us so long as human history lasts. It takes a remarkable faith in human nature to suppose that altruism can become a dominant force in political life when up to this point in history either military force or the power of the profit motive has ensured that maldistributions of resources, basic living conditions and personal liberties can be only marginally altered by appeals to justice and human rights. The politics of love cannot dispense with a doctrine of sin or with a view of how it is to be overcome, that is, a doctrine of salvation.

By way of illustration of such theological ventures in the politics of love I shall refer briefly to two influential accounts of Christian social ethics, firstly that of the Protestant theologian, Reinhold Niebuhr and then that of a group of predominately Roman Catholic writers, the advocates of

Liberation Theology. No attempt will be made to give a full exposition of these richly complex theologies. My summaries will be illustrative only of one cardinal feature, the dialectical nature of the triumph of love in politics, seen as an 'impossible possibility'.

Moral man and immoral society

I take the heading of this section from the title of what is perhaps Niebuhr's best-known book on Christianity and politics. Niebuhr begins from the conviction that sins of pride and concupiscence are a dominant influence in human life and that they are especially evident in social and political life, since it is here that conflicts of interest are at their most extreme. While he accepts that in personal relationships the ideal of self-giving love may have some influence, he believes we must avoid any kind of idealism which supposes that we can eliminate 'the selfish, brutal and antisocial elements, which express themselves in all inter-group life'.[11] Thus, though the individual may have some possibility of acting lovingly, society seems inevitably immoral. This deep-seated suspicion of politics in Niebuhr's writing stems partly from his insistence that Christian love (*agape*) is not to be confused with mutuality. The calculations of justice are designed to achieve mutuality, to equalize advantages in society and eliminate discrimination and disadvantage: but the love which Christianity is founded upon is a self-giving love 'which seeketh not its own', a helping of the other with no thought of return. Niebuhr argues that one cannot base a political policy on such sacrificial love. Politics depends upon balances of *power* which are necessary to neutralize 'the force of egoistic passion' in collective behaviour.

Yet, despite this uncompromising political realism, Niebuhr also believes that 'the impossible ethical ideal'[12] of Christian love *does* have relevance to politics. Here we see a paradoxical strain in his thinking, one which stems from his emphasis on the Cross as both judgement and hope. The closing sentences of his massive study of the doctrine of human nature, *The Nature and Destiny of Man*, contain a memorable summary of this 'dialectic of grace':

Our most reliable understanding is the fruit of 'grace' in which faith completes our ignorance without pretending to possess its certainties as knowledge; and in which contrition mitigates our pride without destroying our hope.[13]

Thus Niebuhr sees love as a necessary 'leaven' in all social and political action, performing both an elevating and a limiting function. This function has effect in three ways: first, by constantly pointing to the 'impossible possibility' of self-giving love, religious faith maintains a passion for the achievement of social justice, which will otherwise be easily lost amidst the harsh realities of social life. Secondly, this impossible possibility negates utopian dreams of human perfectability, because it shows how far short every society falls from a genuinely loving community. Thirdly, this impossible possibility undercuts nationalistic pride by a demand for a love which forgives enemies and draws no boundaries between different human groups.

So the 'impossible ideal' offers at the same time hope and contrition. It encourages us to be constantly seeking for a loving society, in the belief that egoism will not finally prevail. Yet it is always radically critical of any claim to have the final formula for a politics of love. Niebuhr expresses this paradox as follows: 'History moves toward the realisation of the Kingdom, but yet the judgement of God is upon every new realisation.'[14]

Liberation of the oppressed

In many respects the more recent development of various 'political theologies'[15] may be seen as an extension of these ideas of Niebuhr's. There is a similar stress on the idea of the Kingdom of God which must be established on earth, yet whose final form cannot be equated with any human political organization. Like Niebuhr political theologians point to the corruption and greed in human societies and argue that love demands an end to injustice, selfishness and exploitation. But, unlike Niebuhr, most political theologians are quite explicit about the type of political change required if the Kingdom is to be brought closer to reality. This is especially true of those who

121

urge the liberation of the oppressed as the prime aim of Christian love. They tend to stress the 'possible' side of Niebuhr's impossible possibility, arguing for revolutionary change which espouses a clear 'option for the poor'. A very strong statement of this politically partisan love is given by Girardi: 'One must love all, but not all in the same way. One loves the oppressed by liberating them from their misery; one loves the oppressors by liberating them from their sinfulness.'[16] Not all liberation theologians would so readily associate sinfulness only with political oppressors, but they would all argue that the claim of Christianity to liberate one from sin is mere empty abstraction if it has no practical effect in the overcoming of injustice in society. They share an emphasis on the public and communal nature of Christian doctrine. In the words of Vidales, 'The Christian message is not simply a word whispered to individuals in their isolated lives as lone persons.'[17] Indeed the attempt to privatize Christian belief is seen as part of the armoury of oppression, since a salvation which changes only the individual soul poses no threat to those who wield political power to support their privileged position.

It will come as no surprise to learn that liberation theology has frequently seen common ground between Christianity and Marxism,[18] but it must not be supposed that these theologians accept this (or any other political theory) uncritically. Here the 'impossible' side of the impossible possibility reappears. As well as stressing the practical and public aspects of theology, political theologians give theology an unremittingly critical task. There is a powerfully eschatological emphasis in their approach which leads to a stress on the provisional nature of all theological assertions. They look constantly to the 'God of the future' who is bringing about his Kingdom of love on earth. This means that any alignments with specific policies which might be made by them can never be permanent and absolute. If praxis proves such policies to be failing to bring liberation from poverty and oppression, then the political theologian must abandon them for an alternative policy which is closer to the Christian hope for the final Kingdom.

3. LOVE'S EMBODIMENT

At this stage, the substitution of the 'impossible possibilities' of these theologians for the liberal humanism of Titmuss and Watson may scarcely seem much of a gain. Granted the theologians stress the pervasiveness of pride and egoism in communal life, but do they in any sense provide a means of overcoming it? In Niebuhr one finds a tendency to capitulate to what is merely the politics of pragmatism, while in Liberation Theology there often seems an uncritical support of Marxism despite claims to a provisional commitment. But the strength of both approaches lies in their refusal (in theory at least) finally to allow such simple solutions. This refusal is based on an awareness of the uncertain status of all claims to love which do not embody the self-giving love of God revealed in Christ. They require the image of the Church as the body of Christ on earth in order to make concrete and effective their politics of love.

Such an image, however, is easily misinterpreted. It is necessary to make clear that the use of 'the body of Christ' does not imply a Christian triumphalism, which puts Christians in a dominant position as the purveyors of political wisdom and the exemplars of communal love. Such a triumphalist view was promoted by T.S. Eliot in a political pamphlet (the style of which is in dramatic contrast to the subtlety and tentativeness of his poetry), entitled *The Idea of a Christian Society*. In this work Eliot argued that, 'It is only in a society with a religious bias – which is not the same thing as an ecclesiastical despotism – that you can get the proper harmony and tension, for the individual or for the community'.[19] He painted a gloomy picture of the future of a non-religious society, in which, following the inevitable failure of liberal optimism, there would be a decline into mere apathy or a takeover by totalitarianism. It was a bleak prognostication which Auden expressed in his own way in 'The Shield of Achilles':

> A plain without a feature, bare and brown,
>   No blade of grass, no sign of neighbourhood,
> Nothing to eat and nowhere to sit down,

Yet, congregated on its blankness, stood
An unintelligible multitude,
A million eyes, a million boots in line,
Without expression, waiting for a sign.[20]

Against the dangers he foresaw, Eliot offered the bulwark of religious control. Society would require a church within the Church, a group of 'consciously and thoughtfully practising Christians, especially those of intellectual and spiritual superiority'.[21] This Community of Christians would act as 'the conscious mind and consciousness of the nation'.[22] Less thoughtful people would follow their lead.

But the meaning which the image of the body of Christ conveys is precisely the opposite of such spiritual élitism! In the body, all parts, however humble and seemingly unimportant, are equally prized. In the body no member possesses authority and wisdom except that which is given by the head, who is Christ. Moreover, the body of Christ is not characterized by superiority and success, but by vulnerability, humility and failure by worldly standards. It follows that the body of Christ cannot be equated with a group of 'spiritually superior' Christians nor indeed with the institutional churches, when they make exclusivist claims to be that body. The self-confidence of the 'superior Christian' and the outward show of ecclesiastical authority are far removed from the humiliated and despised body of Christ. A living body whose head resolutely seeks love at whatever cost will always be in an unenviable and exposed position. If it remains alive, it is taken into constant danger by its obedience to the head's intentions and commands. It is safe only when it is dead and the head has no more authority over it! Love's body, the Church, seems constantly to die from the sheer impossibility of the demands the head puts upon it – and then to find fresh embodiment in perhaps the same, perhaps another group of people, who try to follow Christ, the incarnation of a total love. In a more perceptive mood, Eliot expressed this fragility of love's hope and persistence in his third quartet, 'The Dry Salvages':

> The hint half guessed, the gift half understood,
>   is Incarnation . . .

Here the past and future
Are conquered, and reconciled

. . . And right action is freedom
From past and future also.
For most of us, this is the aim
Never here to be realised;
Who are only undefeated
Because we have gone on trying;[23]

Love's body goes on trying, sharing a sense of failure, shunning a reputation for love, too deeply aware of how frequently the influence of the past and the lure of the future block the immediacy of incarnate love.

4. THE MODERATION OF LOVE

If 'love's body' is not to be equated with ecclesiastical institutions but with the fellowship of those who keep trying to love, then there is a place in that body for those 'professors of love' who offer help to the sick and disadvantaged as a means of earning a livelihood. (Here, as throughout this book, I am speaking analogically when theological terms are being used. I am not making Christian belief a *sine qua non* of participation in the politics of love. Rather, I am suggesting some 'secular' counterparts to Christian images of transcendent love.) Nevertheless the place offered to the professors may well be a humbler one than they might prefer! We must certainly resist the notion canvassed by Halmos in *The Personal Service Society* that professionals should become culture heroes, the paradigms of loving concern.[24] Such idealization, as I have argued earlier, is quite alien to appropriate professional care. It leads to the elevation of the doctor as 'god' and the nurse as 'angel'. (Social workers, however, rarely suffer from such deceptive projections by their clients.) This elevation obscures the humanity and fallibility of the professional. Yet it is this very humanity which helped persons require in order to receive the grace of a care which gives them value in themselves. To refer back to the argument of the previous chapter, a sacrament ceases to be effective when the earthly material of the sign is confused with that which is signified. Doctors, nurses and social workers are not – as a group at least – heroes and heroines: but a faithful carrying out of their professional tasks does create values which are richer than their inadequate efforts to help. They symbolize transcendent love, when people are at their most vulnerable.

In terms of the politics of love, however, the place of the professions must appear relatively unimportant, though nevertheless necessary. As I have been suggesting throughout this book, what professional carers have to offer to society (in return for the undoubted advantages they receive from it) is the 'moderation of love'. This has been shown to be both a skill (the subtle balance between involvement and detachment) and a symbolic role (the mediation of concern and hope for the individual, even in the most dire illness and distress). But in terms of the politics of love, as I have now defined them by reference to the vulnerability of the body of Christ, professional helpers are far removed from the main action. They are not on the really exposed parts of the vulnerable body, though of course they will perish if the risks of love destroy that body. It is true that the practice of a profession frequently uncovers injustice.[25] But the social position of professionals as moderators protects them from the consequences of their discoveries. They are required to be detached, coolly scientific and not socially disruptive by their very claim to professional status. If they disturb this social compromise (as radical social workers attempt to do without evident success) then they are unlikely to be able to practise their profession in any influential sphere. Mavericks are allowed, of course, but only in limited numbers. To be a moderator is to be prevented by your position from taking sides.

So professionals are apparently somewhat insignificant members of love's body. For, if they risk too much, they are likely to love their supportive and therapeutic function in the body as a whole. Such a conclusion, however, is perhaps too bland. One of the most traumatic reappraisals of professionalism has been provoked by the realization by many members of the medical profession (including those in senior and influential positions) that their professional skill and commitment would be utterly useless in the event of a nuclear war, even one of 'limited' extent.[26] For a profession which sees itself as attempting scientific competence even in the worst conditions this acknowledgement of helplessness is profoundly disturbing. For many doctors it has meant that the politics of nuclear confrontation is no longer *professionally* acceptable. The political issue can no longer be seen as merely a question of personal conviction by some practitioners. Their commitment to medicine requires an abrogation of nuclear war.

This is merely one controversial example, though one which could be seen as the only issue of final significance for the future existence of human life as we know it. But it may indicate the limitations of the moderation of love in professional care. Powerful and beneficial though such balanced and informed expressions of care are, they may be too safe and innocent of political reality to serve love's purposes.

In the previous chapter I saw echoes of Edwin Muir's 'The Transfiguration' in the hopes symbolized by professional care. Perhaps (despite Niebuhr's strictures on nationalism!) I may be permitted to end this exploration of the theology of professional care with another quotation from 'One Foot in Eden' by my fellow Scot. Muir reminds us that the dream of Eden restored may well miss the human condition, for, although innocence cannot be recaptured, love blossoms on the 'famished field and blackened tree' outside Eden:

> But famished field and blackened tree
> Bear flowers in Eden never known.
> Blossoms of grief and charity
> Bloom in these darkened fields alone . . .
>
> Strange blessings never in Paradise
> Fall from these beclouded skies.[27]

Eventually love can *not* be moderate, if it will live in the world after Eden, and professionalism must mean a risky professing, if it will profess love.

Notes

Preamble

1. See J.A. Jackson (ed.), *Professions and Professionalization* (Cambridge 1970); T.J. Johnson, *Professions and Power* (Macmillan 1972); P. Wilding, *Professional Power and Social Welfare* (Routledge and Kegan Paul 1982), ch. 1.

2. The criterion of professional autonomy, which is explained in the next chapter, makes dubious the claims of nurses and social workers to full professional status, and there is also some question of whether their professional practice is based on a clearly defined body of specialist knowledge.

3. An excellent sociological and historical study has been published recently – A. Russell, *The Clerical Profession* (SPCK 1980). I hope to discuss the issue of theology and professionalism, as it relates to pastoral care, in a forthcoming publication (*Pastoral Care and Professionalism*).

1. Lovers and Professors

1. T.S. Eliot, *Complete Poems and Plays* (Faber and Faber 1969), p.98.

2. See Helen Gardner, *The Art of T.S. Eliot* (Faber and Faber 1968), ch.5.

3. For some enjoyable reading on this subject the reader is referred to Malcolm Bradbury, *The History Man* (Arrow Books 1977) and David Lodge, *Changing Places* (Penguin 1978).

4. P. Halmos, *The Personal Service Society* (Constable 1970), p.22.

5. P. Halmos, *The Faith of the Counsellors* (Constable 1965), p.63.

6. Kant puts it as follows: 'For love, as an affection, cannot be commanded, but beneficence for duty's sake may, even though we are not impelled to it by any inclination – nay, are even repelled by a natural and unconquerable aversion.' *Fundamental*

128

Principles of the Metaphysic of Morals (New York, Bobbs Merrill, 1949), p.17.

7. R. Titmuss, *Commitment to Welfare* (Allen and Unwin 1968), p.85.

8. Preface to 'The Doctor's Dilemma', G.B. Shaw, *Collected Plays with their Prefaces*, vol. 3 (The Bodley Head 1971), p.236.

9. See I. Illich, *Limits to Medicine* (Penguin 1977) and *Disabling Professions* (Boyars 1977).

10. Wilding, *Professional Power and Social Welfare*, p.5.

11. ibid., ch.1. These must be seen as *goals* which not all aspiring professions – e.g. social work, nursing – necessarily achieve.

12. Halmos, *The Faith of the Counsellors*, p.3.

13. ibid., p.2.

14. ibid., p.28.

15. ibid., p.175.

16. Halmos, *The Personal Service Society*, p.22. Halmos does not regard his list of personal service professions as exhaustive. In a later part of the book (pp.114–44) he has an interesting discussion of counselling in business management.

17. As Halmos puts it: 'If one wanted to be cynical, one could say that to be a professional is to have one's cake of virtuousness, and also enjoy one's feast of pride and social advantage.' ibid., p.27.

18. See *The Faith of the Counsellors*, pp.74–90. Halmos explicitly acknowledges his sympathy in the Introduction to this book (p.8.), but also claims an objectivity for his account based on the thorough review of literature which has led him to his conclusions. Nevertheless, at least one reviewer felt that the work should be re-titled, 'The Faith of Professor Halmos' (J.A. Mack, *Sociology*, 1968, 2, p.247).

19. Z. Butrym, *The Nature of Social Work* (Macmillan 1976), p.2.

20. P. Halmos, *The Personal and the Political* (Hutchinson 1978), p.15; italics indicate author's emphasis.

21. ibid., p.173.

22. ibid., p.171.

23. Paul Wilding (op.cit., p.12) describes Halmos' theories as speculation 'in a relaxed, post-prandial kind of way', unrelated to any theory of society; Kathleen Jones views *The Personal Service Society* as 'an exercise in social fantasy' (*Sociology*, 1972, 6, p.136).

24. See reviews of *The Personal and the Political* by Geoffrey Pearson (*Brit. J. Soc. Work*, 1978, *8*, p.493) and by David Watson (*J. Social Policy*, 1978, *8*, p.251).

25. Halmos, op. cit., p.182. Similarly, he writes in *The Personal and the Political* (p.20) that 'the *homo religiosus* of the mid-twentieth century hid his faith under the cloak of the personal service professional'.

26. Halmos, op.cit., p.145.

27. See Halmos, *The Personal and the Political*, ch. 7.

28. See J.E. Mayer and N. Timms, *The Client Speaks* (Routledge and Kegan Paul 1970).

29. Gardner, op.cit., p.122.

30. Eliot, *Collected Poems and Plays*, p.180.

31. R. Wilkes, *Social Work with Undervalued Groups* (Tavistock 1981), p.62.

32. ibid., p.88.

2. *Medical Power*

1. E.D. Pellegrino and D.S. Thomasma, *A Philosophical Basis of Medical Practice* (Oxford University Press 1981).

2. T. McKeown, *The Role of Medicine* (The Rock Carling Fellowship, Nuffield Provincial Hospitals Trust, 1976).

3. R. Dubos, *Mirage of Health* (New York, Harper and Row, 1979; first published 1959).

4. See Wilding, *Professional Power and Social Welfare*, especially chapter 2; Eliot Freidson, *Profession of Medicine* (New York, Dodd Mead, 1975); N. Parry and J. Parry, *The Rise of the Medical Profession* (Croom Helm 1976).

5. For a clear and brief summary of this and other sociological theories see T. McGlew and A. Robertson, 'Social Change and the Shifting Boundaries of Discretion in Medicine', in M. Adler and S. Asquith (eds.), *Discretion and Welfare* (Heinemann 1981).

6. See note 4 above.

7. T.J. Johnson, *Professions and Power* (Macmillan 1972), p. 45.

8. Freidson, op.cit., p.82.

9. ibid., pp.27–33.

10. M. Wilson, *Health is for People* (Darton Longman and Todd 1975), p.72.

11. See note 2 above.

12. This point was made with some force by a previous Rock Carling Fellow, A.L. Cochrane in *Effectiveness and Efficiency* (Nuffield Provincial Hospitals Trust 1972).

13. R. Dubos, op.cit.

14. ibid., p.282.

15. Wilson, op.cit., p.77.

16. P. Rhodes, *The Value of Medicine* (Allen and Unwin 1976), p.116.

17. For a brief account of the reconstruction and the full text of the inscription see J.H. Oliver, 'An Ancient Poem on the Duties of a Physician' *Bulletin of the History of Medicine*, 1939, 7, pp.315–23.

18. ibid., p.317f.

19. Preface to 'The Doctor's Dilemma', G.B. Shaw, op. cit., p. 318f.

20. Leo Tolstoy, *The Death of Ivan Ilyich*, (Penguin 1960), p.126.

21. See L. Edelstein, *Ancient Medicine: Selected Papers*, edited by O. Temkin and C.L. Temkin (Baltimore, Johns Hopkins, 1967).

22. Quoted in M. Foucault, *The Birth of the Clinic: An Archaeology of Medical Perception*, translated by A.M. Sheridan Smith (Tavistock 1973), p.88.

23. See A.V. Campbell and R. Higgs, *In That Case: Medical Ethics in Everyday Practice* (Darton Longman and Todd 1982), ch.3, for a discussion of the 'professional manner'.

24. Foucault, p.146 (see note 22 above).

25. ibid., p.195.

26. R. Lambourne, 'Towards an Understanding of Medico-Theological Dialogue', in M.A.H. Melinsky (ed.), *Religion and Medicine* 2 (SCM 1973), pp.12–23.

27. A. Siirala, *The Voice of Illness: A Study in Therapy and Prophecy* (Philadelphia, Fortress Press, 1964), p.84.

28. A. Sexton, *The Awful Rowing Toward God* (Boston, Houghton Mifflin, 1975), pp.74f.

29. However, there is scholarly disagreement about the meaning of this precept, and some would dispute this type of explanation. For a different account see Edelstein, op.cit. (note 21 above).

30. P. Lain Entralgo, *Doctor and Patient* (World University Library 1969), p.23.

31. Plato, *Laws*, 720. See Lain Entralgo, op.cit., pp.30–6.

32. Pellegrino and Thomasma, op.cit., p.80.

33. Siirala, op.cit., p.136.

34. M. Balint, *The Doctor, The Patient and His Illness*, 2nd edn (Pitman 1964).

35. See I. Illich, *Limits to Medicine* (Penguin 1977), especially Part 4.

3. Nursing, Nurturing and Sexism

1. In an address given in 1897 to graduating nurses at Johns Hopkins Hospital, quoted in Janet Muff (ed.), *Socialisation, Sexism and Stereotyping: Women's Issues in Nursing* (Mosby 1982), p.215.

2. B. Ehrenreich and D. English, *Witches, Midwives and Nurses: A History of Women Healers* (Writers and Readers Publishing Co-operative, 14 Talacre Road, London, 1973), p.59.

3. I.D. Suttie, *The Origins of Love and Hate* (Kegan Paul, Trench, Trubner, 1935), p.83.

4. 'Nursing as a Profession for Ladies', *St Paul's Monthly Magazine*, August 1871, quoted in B. Abel-Smith, *A History of the Nursing Profession* (Heinemann 1960), p.18.

5. Abel-Smith, op.cit., p.67.

6. See 'Some thoughts on being a male in nursing' by G. Brookfield *et al.* in Muff (ed.), op.cit., pp. 273–7.

7. For a comprehensive, but admirably brief, summary of recent research see M.B. Sutherland, *Sex Bias in Education* (Blackwell 1981), ch.3.

8. In this context, the career success of men in English nursing, now that they have equal opportunities, is illuminating: although only approximately 17% of nurses in England are male, between 40% and 50% of senior positions in administration and nursing education are now held by men. See P. Nuttall, 'Male Takeover or Female Giveaway?', *Nursing Times*, 12 January, 1983, p.10f.

9. The high awareness in the USA about sexism in medicine and nursing can be easily understood when we notice the marked sexual polarization in the two professions there: not only are 92% of American doctors male, 98% or even 99% of American nurses are female. See Ehrenreich and English, op.cit.; Muff (ed.), op.cit.

10. 'Toward Androgeny', in Muff (ed.), op.cit., p.253.

11. E. Whittaker and V. Oleson in R. Dingwall and J. MacKintosh (eds.), *Readings in the Sociology of Nursing* (Churchill Livingstone 1978), p.26.

12. ibid., p.23. See *The Writings of Henry Wadsworth Longfellow*, vol. 5 (Routledge 1886), p.53.

13. Quoted in Abel-Smith, op.cit., p.27.

14. ibid., p.99.

15. R. White, *Social Change and the Development of the Nursing Profession* (Kimpton 1978).

16. These quotations are cited in Margaret Connor Veruysen's paper: 'Old Wives Tales? Women Healers in English History', in Celia Davies (ed.), *Rewriting Nursing History* (Croom Helm 1980), p.182.

17. K. Kesey, *One Flew Over the Cuckoo's Nest* (Picador 1973), p.27.

18. This summary of Hall's theory is based on the account given in B.J. Stevens, *Nursing Theory: Analysis, Application, Evaluation* (Boston, Little Brown, 1979), ch.2.

19. D.E. Orem, *Nursing: Concepts of Practice* (New York, McGraw Hill, 1971), p.69.

20. ibid., p.78.

21. For a helpful overview of four such theories (including Orem's) see E.A. McFarlane, *Journal of Advanced Nursing*, 1980, 5, pp.3–19; and for a thorough critique of the nature of nursing theory see Barbara J. Stevens, op.cit. (note 18 above).

22. Stevens, op.cit., p.93.

23. K. Williams, 'Ideologies of Nursing: their meanings and implications', *Nursing Times*, 70 (8 August 1974), Occasional Paper.

24. May Clark, 'Getting through the work', in Dingwall and MacKintosh, op.cit., pp.67–86 (see note 11 above).

25. F. Stockwell, *The Unpopular Patient* (RCN and National Council of Nurses of the UK 1972).

26. Clark, op.cit., p.77.

27. ibid.

28. ibid.

29. ibid., p.80.

30. ibid.

31. The poem is quoted (at greater length) in Mick Carpenter, 'Asylum Nursing Before 1914: a Chapter in the History of Labour', in C. Davies, op.cit., p.141f.

32. Stockwell, op.cit., p.54.

33. See the summary of similar studies in Stockwell, op.cit., ch.13.
34. ibid., p.47.
35. J. Vanier, *Tears of Silence* (Darton Longman and Todd 1973), p.25.
36. Stevens, op.cit., p.228 (see note 18 above).
37. I have already explored this concept in a previous work – *Rediscovering Pastoral Care* (Darton Longman and Todd 1981), ch.7 – but in that discussion I had a non-professional context in mind, in which faith was the main issue. My use of it in the context of nursing has a less explicit (but no less deliberate) reference to faith.

4. *The Two Faces of Social Work*

1. Z. Butrym, *The Nature of Social Work* (Macmillan 1976), p.12.
2. B. Reynolds, 'Between Client and Community: a Study of Responsibility in Social Casework', *Smith College Studies in Social Work*, vol. 5, no. 1 (1934), p.125.
3. J.E. Mayer and N. Timms, *The Client Speaks* (Routledge and Kegan Paul 1970), p.69.
4. In the U.K. Scotland differs from England and Wales in this respect, the latter countries having retained a separate Probation Service in the reorganization of social work services, while Scotland has not.
5. See *The Social Work Task* (British Association of Social Workers 1977).
6. ibid., p.19, para. 3.17.
7. A. Pincus and A. Minahan, *Social Work Practice: Model and Method* (Itasca, Illinois, Peacock Publishers, 1975), p.9.
8. The reference to Lincoln's Gettysburg Address is mine, not the authors'.
9. Butrym, op.cit., ch.2.
10. *The Social Work Task*, p.18, para. 3.16.
11. N. Ragg, *People not Cases* (Routledge and Kegan Paul 1977).
12. R. Wilkes, *Social Work with Undervalued Groups* (Tavistock 1981).
13. ibid., p.80.
14. ibid., p.62.

15. Ragg, op.cit., p.78.
16. D. Statham, *Radicals in Social Work* (Routledge and Kegan Paul 1978), p.35.
17. P. Corrigan and P. Leonard, *Social Work Practice Under Capitalism* (Macmillan 1978), p.123.
18. J. Galper, *The Politics of Social Services* (Englewood Cliffs, New Jersey, Prentice Hall, 1975), p.142.
19. See R. Bailey and M. Brake (eds.), *Radical Social Work* (Edward Arnold 1975) p.147.
20. Galper, op.cit., p.45.
21. Corrigan and Leonard, op.cit., p.155.
22. Statham, op.cit., p.10.
23. Galper, op.cit., p.189.
24. Corrigan and Leonard, op.cit., p.154.
25. Galper, op.cit., pp.226f.
26. ibid., p.189.
27. Corrigan and Leonard, op.cit., p.157.
28. Wilkes, op.cit., p.101.
29. See Halmos, *The Personal and the Political: Social Work and Political Action* (Hutchinson 1978), ch.6.
30. G. Pearson, *The Deviant Imagination* (Macmillan 1975), p.132.
31. ibid., p.129.
32. See, for example, P. Wilding, *Professional Power and Social Welfare* (Routledge and Kegan Paul 1982), ch.1 and P. Leonard 'The Function of Social Work in Society: A preliminary exploration' in N. Timms and D. Watson (eds.), *Talking about Welfare: Readings in Philosophy and Social Policy* (Routledge and Kegan Paul 1976).
33. See Leonard, op.cit.
34. ibid., p.263. Leonard himself seems undecided between the mediation model and the adversary model, but tends in his later writing to favour the latter.
35. W.B. Yeats, *Collected Poems* (Macmillan 1960), p.184.
36. 'A Paradigm for Radical Practice', in Bailey and Brake (eds.), op.cit., p.53.
37. Ragg, op.cit., p.75.

38. F.P. Biestek, *The Casework Relationship* (Allen and Unwin 1967).

39. See 'A Critique of the Principle of Client Self-Determination', in F.E. McDermott (ed.), *Self-Determination in Social Work* (Routledge and Kegan Paul 1975), ch.3.

40. ibid., chs. 2, 5 and 6.

41. Wilkes, op.cit., p.16.

42. See David Soyer, 'The Right to Fail', McDermott (ed.), op.cit., ch.4.

43. W.H. Auden, *Selected Poems* (Faber and Faber 1968), p.78.

5. The Claim to Purity

1. See E. Fromm, *Man for Himself* (Routledge and Kegan Paul 1948), *passim*.

2. E. Fromm, *Psychoanalysis and Religion* (Gollancz 1951). See also J. Hillman, *Insearch* (Hodder and Stoughton 1967), ch.1.

3. *Man for Himself*, p.129.

4. See R.S. Downie and E. Telfer, *Respect for Persons* (Allen and Unwin 1969); and G. Outka, *Agape: An Ethical Analysis* (New Haven, Yale U.P., 1972).

5. E. Fromm, *The Art of Loving* (Allen and Unwin 1972), p.38.

6. ibid., p.25.

7. P. Tillich, *Love, Power and Justice* (Oxford U.P. 1954; Galaxy edn 1960), p.26.

8. The link here is Tillich's concept of 'being-itself', which equally describes love and God. See P. Tillich, *Systematic Theology*, vol. 1 (Nisbet 1968), p. 310.

9. See A. Nygren, *Agape and Eros* (SPCK 1953).

10. P. Tillich, *Morality and Beyond* (Harper and Row 1963), p.89.

11. M. Scheler, *The Nature of Sympathy*, translated by Peter Heath (Routledge and Kegan Paul 1954), p.5.

12. ibid., p.12.

13. Scheler refers to the work of Le Bon and of Freud (*Group Psychology and the Analysis of the Ego*) in this context.

14. See especially Scheler's discussion of 'the sympathetic functions' in *The Nature of Sympathy*, Part I, ch.7.

15. ibid., p.35, author's emphases.

16. ibid., p.46, author's emphases.

17. ibid., p.161.

18. ibid., p.70, from Tagore's poem, 'The Gardener'.

19. K. Gibran, *The Prophet* (Heinemann 1976), p.19.

20. L. Edelstein, 'The Hippocratic Oath: Text, Translation and Interpretation,' in O. Temkin and C.L. Temkin (eds.), *Ancient Medicine* (Baltimore, Johns Hopkins, 1967), p.62f.

21. Brian Abel-Smith describes the uniform of lady-pupils in the Middlesex Hospital after the Nightingale reform: 'they were resplendent in a dress of violet hue with a small train, three inches in length, which swept the floor behind them'. The purpose of the train was made evident by the matron, Mrs Thorold, when a delinquent dared to turn up her frayed hem: 'I will not allow it to be done, dear. I devised this little train so that when you lean over a bed to attend a patient your ankles will be covered and the students will not be able to see them.' *A History of the Nursing Profession* (Heinemann 1960), p.31, note 7.

22. B. Ehrenreich and D. English, *Witches, Midwives and Nurses: A History of Women Healers* (Writers and Readers Publishing Co-operative 1973), p.61.

23. See Abel-Smith, op.cit., p.114.

24. ibid., ch.8, *passim*.

25. *Collected Essays, Journalism and Letters of George Orwell*, vol.4 (Penguin 1970).

26. R. Wilkes, *Social Work with Undervalued Groups* (Tavistock 1981), p.53.

27. A. Flexner, 'Is Social Work a Profession?' in *Proceedings of the National Conference of Charities and Correction* (Chicago, Hildmann Printing Company, 1915), p.590.

28. See R. Niebuhr, *An Interpretation of Christian Ethics* (SCM 1936).

29. 'The Transfiguration', *Collected Poems of Edwin Muir* (Faber and Faber 1963), p.200.

6. Knowing What is Best

1. E. Hughes, *Men and Their Work* (Glencoe, Illinois, Free Press, 1958).

2. R.D. Laing, *Knots* (Penguin Books 1970).

3. Louis MacNeice, *Collected Poems*, edited by E.R. Dodds (Faber and Faber 1966), p.193.

4. T.S. Eliot, 'Preludes', *Collected Poems 1909–1935* (Faber and Faber 1957), p.22.

5. For a modern rendering of this famous passage (and the rest of the text of the revelations) see *Revelations of Divine Love*, translated by C. Wolters (Penguin Classics 1966), p.211.

6. 'Code, Covenant, Contract or Philanthropy', *The Hastings Center Report*, vol.5, no.6 (December 1975), p.37.

7. See *The Knowledge of Man*, edited by M. Friedman (Allen and Unwin 1965), Appendix.

8. M. Scheler, *The Nature of Sympathy* (Routledge and Kegan Paul 1954), Part 2, ch.3.

9. K. Browne and P. Freeling, *The Doctor-Patient Relationship* (Churchill Livingstone 1976), p.62.

10. J. Mathers in M.A.H. Melinsky (ed.), *Religion and Medicine: A Discussion* (SCM 1970), p.8.

11. See A.H. Maslow, *Motivation and Personality* (Harper and Row 1954).

12. Such ideas tend to be relegated to the 'lunatic fringe' by professional groups. Yet, from another perspective the impoverished setting in which professionals practise could be regarded as the 'fringe'. The culture of medicine and nursing creates a bare clinical environment and of social work an equally denuded office setting. Such environments appear to deny any goodness to the natural world.

13. D.D. Williams, *The Spirit and the Forms of Love* (Nisbet 1968), p.3.

14. George Herbert, 'Prayer', *Faber Book of Religious Verse*, edited by H. Gardner (Faber and Faber 1979), p.122.

15. See R.A. Lambourne, *Community, Church and Healing* (Darton Longman and Todd 1963), ch.7.

16. The idea of the hospital as a 'temple of humanism' was expressed in an article by Robert Lambourne in the context of hospital chaplaincy. See 'The Hospital as a Source of Standards and Values', *Contact*, 16 (January 1966).

7. Caring and Being Cared For

1. J. Hillman, *Insearch* (Hodder and Stoughton 1967), p.13.

2. *Oxford Book of Contemporary Verse*, 1945–1980, chosen by D.J. Enright (Oxford U.P. 1980), p.81.

3. D.D. Williams, op. cit., p.288.

4. P. Ramsey, *The Patient as Person* (Yale U.P. 1970), p.xii, author's emphasis.

5. ibid.

6. W.F. May, 'Code, Covenant, Contract or Philanthropy', in *The Hastings Center Report*, vol.5 (December 1975), pp.29–38. Although this refers specifically to medicine, May's ideas can be applied more widely. See also his recent publication, *Physician's Covenant: Images of the Healer in Medical Ethics* (Westminster Press 1983).

7. W.F. May, 'Code, Covenant, Contract or Philanthropy', p.34.

8. ibid., p.30.

9. Hillman, op.cit., ch.1.

10. H.A. Eadie, 'The Helping Personality', *Contact*, 49 (Summer 1975), pp.2–17.

11. Excerpts from 'He's frightfully good at coping' by Paris Leary from *Poets of Today*, *VII*, (New York, Scribner, 1960).

12. No doubt this is an interpretation of the text, which may be reading more into it than is justified. Yet the striking physical descriptions in this story can scarcely be ignored. As in other similar stories, the actions are as important as the words which accompany them. It is unfortunate that subsequent tradition has put the emphasis on the woman's sinfulness and (through a confusion with Mary Magdalene, who is mentioned in the subsequent chapter) has created 'maudlin' associations of a weeping penitent woman saved from sexual sin. This is more the attitude of the Pharisee than that of Jesus!

13. E. Moltmann-Wendel, *The Women Around Jesus* (SCM 1982), p.102.

14. See I.D. Suttie, *The Origins of Love and Hate* (Kegan Paul, Trench and Trubner 1935), ch.6. A striking example of such care is described in John Steinbeck's *Grapes of Wrath*, when a young mother suckles a weak, dying old man.

15. See the conclusion to chapter 5 above.

8. The Politics of Love

1. W.H. Auden, *Selected Poems* (Faber and Faber 1968), p.78.
2. D.D. Williams, *The Spirit and the Forms of Love*, p.243.
3. Edwin Muir, *Collected Poems* (Faber and Faber 1963), p.227.
4. A book of this title by J. Ferguson (James Clarke 1973) deals with Christian pacifism rather than with the wider topic of this chapter.
5. R. Titmuss, *The Gift Relationship* (Allen and Unwin 1970), p.212.
6. ibid., p.242.
7. D. Watson, *Caring for Strangers* (Routledge and Kegan Paul 1980).
8. K.E. Boulding, 'The Boundaries of Social Policy' *Social Work* (USA), vol. 12, no. 1.
9. D.D. Williams, op.cit., p.243.
10. See note 3 above.
11. R. Niebuhr, *Moral Man and Immoral Society* (New York, Scribner, 1932), p.75.
12. R. Niebuhr, *An Interpretation of Christian Ethics* (SCM 1936), p.150.
13. R. Niebuhr, *The Nature and Destiny of Man*, vol. 2 (Nisbet 1943), p.332.
14. ibid., p.296.
15. For an admirable summary and critique of these theologies see A. Fierro, *The Militant Gospel* (SCM 1977).
16. Quoted in Fierro, op.cit., p.191.
17. R. Vidales in R. Gibellini (ed.), *Frontiers of Theology in Latin America* (SCM 1980), p.53.
18. See especially J.P. Miranda, *Marx and the Bible* (SCM 1977).
19. T.S. Eliot, *The Idea of a Christian Society* (Faber and Faber 1938), p.42.
20. Auden, *Selected Poems*, p.78 (see note 1 above).
21. Eliot, op.cit., p.35.
22. ibid., p.42.
23. *Complete Poems and Plays of T.S. Eliot* (Faber and Faber 1969), p.190.

24. See P. Halmos, *The Personal Service Society* (Constable 1970), ch.2.

25. A recent example of this uncovering is a report of a British government working party into social inequality and health, which met under the chairmanship of Sir Douglas Black, President of the Royal College of Physicians of London. See P. Townsend and N. Davidson (eds.), *Inequalities in Health: The Black Report* (Penguin 1982).

26. *Report of the Board of Science and Education Inquiry into the Medical Effects of Nuclear War* (British Medical Association 1983).

27. Edwin Muir, op. cit.

Select Bibliography

The following brief selection, taken largely from works cited in the list of references, is designed to guide the reader towards major works in the various fields under discussion in this book. More information can be obtained by following up the detailed references given for each chapter, or by consulting bibliographies given in the works listed below.

1. Professions and Social Welfare

Adler, M. and Asquith, S. (eds.), *Discretion and Welfare*. Heinemann 1981.
Halmos, P., *The Faith of the Counsellors*. Constable 1965.
Halmos, P., *The Personal Service Society*. Constable 1970.
Halmos, P., *The Personal and the Political*. Hutchinson 1978.
Illich, I., *Disabling Professions*. Boyars 1977.
Johnson, T.J., *Professions and Power*. Macmillan 1972.
Wilding, P., *Professional Power and Social Welfare*. Routledge and Kegan Paul 1982.

2. Medicine and Health

Dubos, R., *Mirage of Health: Utopias, Progress and Biological Change*. New York, Harper and Row, 1959.
Foucault, M., *The Birth of the Clinic: An Archaeology of Medical Perception*. Tavistock 1973.
Freidson, E., *Profession of Medicine*. New York, Dodd Mead, 1975.
Lambourne, R.A., *Community, Church and Healing*. Darton Longman and Todd 1963.
McKeown, T., *The Role of Medicine: Dream, Mirage or Nemesis?* Nuffield Provincial Hospitals Trust 1976.
Pellegrino, E.D., and Thomasma, D.C. *A Philosophical Basis of Medical Practice*. Oxford U.P. 1981.

Siirala, A., *The Voice of Illness: A Study in Therapy and Prophecy*, Philadelphia, Fortress Press, 1964.
Wilson, M., *Health is for People*. Darton Longman and Todd 1975.

3. Nursing, Theory and Practice

Abel-Smith, B., *A History of the Nursing Profession*. Heinemann 1960.
Davies, C. (ed.), *Rewriting Nursing History*. Croom Helm 1980.
Dingwall, R. and McIntosh, J. (eds.), *Readings in the Sociology of Nursing*. Churchill Livingstone 1978.
Muff, J. (ed.), *Socialization, Sexism and Stereotyping: Women's Issues in Nursing*. Mosby 1982.
Stevens, B.J., *Nursing Theory: Analysis, Application, Evaluation*. Boston, Little Brown, 1979.
Stockwell, F., *The Unpopular Patient*. Royal College of Nursing 1972.
White, R. *Social Change and the Development of the Nursing Profession: A Study of the Poor Law Nursing Service 1848–1948*. Henry Kimpton 1978.

4. Social Work – Personal and Political

Butrym, Z.T., *The Nature of Social Work*. Macmillan 1976.
Corrigan, P. and Leonard, P., *Social Work Practice under Capitalism: A Marxist Approach*. Macmillan 1978.
Galper, J.H., *The Politics of Social Services*. Englewood Cliffs, New Jersey, Prentice Hall, 1975.
Pearson, G., *The Deviant Imagination: Psychiatry, Social Work and Social Change*. Macmillan 1975.
Pincus, A. and Minahan, A., *Social Work Practice: Model and Method*. Itasca, Illinois, Peacock Publishers, 1975.
Plant, R., *Social and Moral Theory in Casework*. Routledge and Kegan Paul 1970.
Ragg, N.M., *People Not Cases: A Philosophical Approach to Social Work*. Routledge and Kegan Paul 1977.
Timms, N. and Watson, D., *Talking about Welfare: Readings in Philosophy and Social Policy*. Routledge and Kegan Paul 1976.
Titmuss, R., *The Gift Relationship*. Allen and Unwin 1970.
Wilkes, R., *Social Work with Undervalued Groups*. Tavistock 1981.

5. *The Nature of Love*

D'Arcy, M.C., *The Mind and the Heart of Love*. Collins Fontana 1962.

Fromm, E., *The Art of Loving*. Allen and Unwin 1972.

Lewis, C.S., *The Four Loves*. Collins Fontana 1960.

McIntyre, J., *On the Love of God*. Collins 1962.

Nygren, A., *Agape and Eros*. SPCK 1953.

Outka, G., *Agape: An Ethical Analysis*. New Haven, Yale U.P., 1972.

Scheler, M., *The Nature of Sympathy* (trans. P. Heath). Routledge and Kegan Paul, 1954.

Tillich, P., *Love, Power and Justice*. Oxford U.P. 1954.

Williams, D.D., *The Spirit and the Forms of Love*. Nisbet 1968.

Index

Abel-Smith, Brian   36, 40, 132, 133
acceptance   74, 108, 112
'action system'   54, 55
Adler, M. and Asquith, S.   130
adversary model   63
aetiology   21; of alcoholism   18
agape   13, 32, 72, 73, 74, 81–5, 114, 120
ageing   95
aggression   37
'alienist'   29
altruism   9, 11, 12, 71, 74, 77–83, 88, 116–19
American Medical Association   20; code of ethics of   24
American National Association of Social Workers code of ethics   78
Anatomy of Human Destructiveness, The   72
ancient symbols   68, 105
ancillary health workers   1
'androgeny'   38
angel of mercy   35, 39, 125
anointing   101, 108, 109; by a sinful woman   108; for burial   109
anxiety   29, 37, 72, 74, 106, 108, 112
'aphasic'   44
'apostolic function' of doctors   31
architecture   97
archetypal symbols   105
arousal, sexual   110
art   70, 78
Art of Loving, The   71
art of nursing   43
arthritis   48, 106
Asclepius   21, 22, 31
Ash Wednesday   14, 15, 49
Asquith, S., Adler, M. and   130
associations, professional   83
'assumptive world'   93, 96
asylums   79
Auden, W.H.   68, 115, 123, 136, 140
authority   92, 124; doctor's   26, 40; medical   18, 19, 24, 25, 37; professional   2

autonomy   19, 42, 61, 111
awareness   77, 108, 110

Bacon, Francis   21
Bailey, R. and Brake, M.   135
Balint, Michael   31, 132
'basic gifts'   118
'basic nursing tasks'   41
bedridden patients   109
behaviour   72, 120; crowd   76
being 'managed'   108
'being present'   92
'being with'   35, 45, 48, 50
belief   10; Christian   98; religious   14
believer   85, 94
betrayal   86, 103
Bichat   25
Biestek, F.P.   65, 136
bilateral transfer   117
Birth of the Clinic, The   25
blood donation   117, 118
bodily integrity   29, 111
body of Christ   123, 124, 126
body expert   39, 43, 90
body language   99
Boulding, K.E.   117, 140
Bradbury, Malcolm   128
Brake, M., Bailey, R. and   135
Britain   38, 79, 118
British Abortion Act   18
British Association of Social Workers (BASW)   53, 54, 55, 63, 64
British Medical Journal   40
Brookfield, G.   132
brother, doctor as   22f.
brotherliness   26, 27f., 70, 111, 114
Brown K. and Freeling, P.   138
Buber, Martin   92
burial   109f.
Butrym, Zofia   52, 55, 129, 134

Campbell, A.V. and Higgs, R.   131
Canadian Nursing Association code of ethics   49
capitalism   57–63

145

Index

care and caring 101ff., 111f., *et passim*
Caring for Strangers 117
Carpenter, Mick 133
Case Con 58
case-work 15, 52, 56, 57, 61, 65, 66, 82, 113
case-work relationship 65
Causley, Charles 101, 105
celebration 99, 108
change-agent (system) 54, 55, 60, 113
charisma(ta) 107
charity 54, 115, 119, 127
Christ 74, 86, 89, 117, 123, 124
'Christ the Recrucified' 111
Christian belief 98, 122, 125; doctrine 91; humanism 95; images 125; love 120, 122; social ethics 119; symbolism 86, 90; theology 88, 95; triumphalism 123
Church 93, 123, 124; government 84
civilization 22; diseases of 97
claim to purity 12, 70ff.
Clark, May 45, 48, 49, 133
class 57–9, 62, 63, 79, 96
clergy 2, 8, 9, 106, 113
client: participation 65; self-determination 65, 96; system 54, 55
clinical psychology 8
closeness 50, 110, 111
Cochrane, A. L. 131
code of ethics 6, 7; of the American Medical Association 24; of the Canadian Nursing Association 49; of the National Association of Social Workers (USA) 70; for Radical Social Service Workers 60
College of Nursing 36, 79
Commitment to Welfare 6
community 8, 21, 30, 45, 84, 97, 99, 111, 117, 121, 123, 124; development 9; health care 18; work 65
companionship 50, 51, 70, 88, 110, 111f.
competitiveness 84, 116, 118
conceptual framework 43f.
conflict 62, 63; model 64
connectedness 95f, 98
consensus 62
consent 28
contract 102f.
control model 63
Corrigan, P. and Leonard, P. 57, 59, 60, 135

counselling 8, 9, 29, 65
counsellor 8–11
'courage to be' 74
covenant 102f., 111
creation 89, 95f, 117
critical distance 81
cross, the 90, 111, 120
'crucified God' 90
crucifixion 85, 88
culture heroes 9, 125

Davidson, N., Townsend, P. and 141
Davies, Celia 133
death 18, 20, 25, 26, 29, 30, 50, 51, 82, 85, 95, 96, 109, 124
Death of Ivan Ilyich, The 23
dedication 40, 70, 71, 78, 79, 83, 105
'defensive over-treatment' 104
definitions: of alcoholism 18; of health 21; of social work 53
degradation 42, 50, 82
demanding patient 48, 50
democracy 60, 62
dependence 90, 92, 96, 112
desire 73–5, 78, 80
detachment 82, 83, 85, 90, 105, 126
diagnosis 44, 56, 90, 91, 94
'dialectic of grace' 120
dietary habits 97
differences, sexual 37, 38
difficult patient 48, 50
dignity 70, 73, 77
dimensions of hope 53, 64, 67f, 113f.
Dingwall, R. and MacKintosh, J. 132, 133
disability 17, 20, 30, 31, 53, 81, 105, 109, 116
disadvantaged 62, 63, 81, 85, 106, 116, 120, 125
discipline 40, 82, 92
discrimination 35, 36, 120
disease 17, 20–2, 25, 26, 80, 90, 91, 94, 98
disease eradication 94, 111
diseases of civilization 97
distress 28, 35, 65, 76, 80, 82, 90, 126
distribution of wealth, power and status 7, 63, 119
doctor as God and as brother 22f, 125
doctor–patient relationship 17, 22, 27, 28
Dodds, E.R. 138
'doing to' 35, 45, 48, 50
dominance 72, 76, 78, 90, 97, 112;

Index

maternal 42; medical 18f, 32; of women 39
Downie, R.S. and Telfer, E. 136
dreams 20ff, 89, 127
'Dry Salvages, The' 124
Dubos, René 17, 21, 33, 98, 130, 131

Eadie, Hugh A. 106, 139
economics 19, 62, 65, 104, 117–19
ecstasy 76, 89
Edelstein, Ludwig 78, 131, 137
Eden 21, 86, 98, 111, 127
education 37, 65, 92, 117
egalitarianism 92
egoism 7, 9, 12, 19, 71, 74, 77, 80, 83, 88, 114, 120, 121, 123
Ehrenreich, B. and English, D. 34, 79, 132, 137
Einfühlung 75, 76, 81
Einsfühlung 75, 76, 81
Eliot, T.S. 5, 14, 15, 16, 49, 88, 123, 124, 128, 130, 138, 140
élitism 79, 124
emotion 6, 11, 28, 35, 37, 38, 41, 48, 66, 72, 73, 74, 75, 76, 77, 81, 82, 85, 105, 108, 110
'emotional women' 35
empathy 9, 37, 75–7, 81, 82
'enabling' 44, 67, 78
encounter 13, 48, 91, 92, 105
English, D., Ehrenreich, B. and 34, 79, 132, 137
enhancement 54, 77, 82, 83, 85, 118
Enright, D.J. 139
environment 20, 21, 25, 29, 37, 48, 53, 54, 64, 68, 76, 96
epithymia 73, 74, 79f, 111
eros 73, 74, 79–81, 114
estrangement 73, 74
eternity 25, 73
ethical codes 5, 6, 7, 78
ethics 6, 8, 13, 17, 19, 53, 59, 71, 74, 75, 81, 83, 119; medical 20, 102
ethos, professional 81, 82, 96
existence 74, 83, 98
existentialism 48, 92
experience 74, 76, 82, 92, 93, 98
expertise 83, 89, 90, 101
exploitation 57, 58, 79, 103, 108, 121

'Faces of Florence Nightingale, The' 39
failure 53, 124, 125
faith 8–11, 14, 15, 74, 89, 90, 93, 94, 98, 99, 101, 119, 121; absurdity of 14

Faith of the Counsellors, The 7, 8, 11, 13
faithfulness 70, 102, 114
fallibility 85, 95, 125
'false consciousness' 57, 90
false piety 83
family 53, 54, 63, 96, 113, 117
family doctor 18
fear 20, 30, 32, 41
Fear of Freedom, The 72
feelings 75, 77, 81
fellow-feeling 71f., 75–7, 81, 114
female, feminine 34, 36–8, 39, 44, 79
Ferguson, J. 140
ferocious goodwill 101, 105
fidelity 102, 104, 105
Fierro, A. 140
Flexner, Abraham 83, 137
foolishness (of faith) 98–101
fore-telling 30
forth-telling 30
Foucault, Michel 25, 131
Four Quartets 15
Francis, St 116
freedom 98, 108, 118, 119, 125
Freeling, P., Brown, K. and 138
Freud, Sigmund 20, 99, 136
Friedman, M. 138
Friedson, Eliot 19, 79, 85, 130
friend, friendship 30, 32, 49, 50, 73, 74, 81, 82, 85, 111
Fromm, Erich 71, 72, 73, 74, 75, 80, 83, 136
fulfilment 51, 97, 107
furor therapeuticus 31
future 113, 122, 125; hope 14; orientation 38; prediction of 30

Galper, Jeffrey 58, 59, 60, 135
Gardner 5, 14, 128, 138
Geary Dean, Patricia 38
General Register of Nurses 79
geriatrics 30, 31, 47, 50
germ theory of disease 21
Gibellini, R., Vidales, R. and 140
Gibran, Khalil 78, 137
gift 103, 105, 107, 117, 124
gift relationship 116, 117f.
Girardi 122
God 22, 70, 73, 74, 87, 90, 91, 93, 94, 98, 103, 106, 111, 121–3, 125
godlikeness 23f., 25, 26, 32, 34
government 19, 84, 85
grace 8, 74, 102, 107, 120, 121, 125

147

gracefulness 107, 108, 110f.
gratitude 106f., 114
gratuitousness 103–6, 114
groups 55, 63, 71, 76, 79, 83, 103, 111
growth 72, 96, 97, 101, 103

Hall, Lydia E. 43, 44, 46, 133
Halmos, Paul 6, 7, 8, 9, 10, 11, 12, 13, 14, 60, 61, 64, 115, 125, 128, 129, 130, 135, 141
'handmaiden' 110
hatred 9, 77, 85
healers 17; women 79
healing 25, 99, 105
healing words 30
health care policy 116
health, definitions of 21; denying 111, 112; education 92
Health is for People 20, 21
health and welfare services 1, 18
Heath, Peter 136
'Helping Personality, The' 106
Herbert, George 99, 138
heroes, health workers as 39, 109, 111, 125, 126
Higgs, R., Campbell, A.V. and 131
Hillman, James 101, 105, 136, 139
Hippocrates, Oath of 70, 78, 79
Hippocratic *Precepts* 27
Hippocratic writings 24
history 20, 74, 93, 94, 115, 119, 121
history of social work 113
Hobbes, Thomas 20
holiness 70, 78, 79, 99
hope 28, 53, 64, 113 *et passim*
hopefulness 70, 111f., 114
hospital 18, 41, 45, 47, 80, 94, 99
How the Poor Die 80
Hughes, Everett 87, 137
humanism 60, 95, 123
Hume, David 72, 75
Hygieia 21, 31
Hymn of Serapion 22, 79

Idea of a Christian Society, The 123
idealism 5, 120
identification 75–7, 81, 90, 92, 114
Illich, Ivan 6, 31, 129, 132
images 61, 79, 88, 111, 113, 119, 123–5
impossible possibilities 119f, 123
incarnation 85, 89, 90, 91, 95, 98, 124
incarnate knowledge 29–32, 88
incompleteness 90, 93f.
injustice 63, 68, 84, 113, 121, 122, 126

Insearch 105
institutionalization 94
integrity 9, 70, 78; bodily 29, 31, 111
inter-personal relationships 53–5
intervention 26, 31, 55f., 66, 90
I-thou relationship 92

Janus 52
Jaspers, Carl 77, 82
Jesus 74, 89, 108, 109, 110
Johnson, T.A. 19, 128, 130
Jones, Kathleen 129
joy 76, 98, 99
Judas 86, 112
judgement 82, 89, 104, 120
Julian of Norwich 89
justice 11, 12f., 53, 63, 114, 115, 119–21

Kant, Immanuel 6, 72, 128
Kantian ethics 57, 75
Kazantzakis, Nikos 89
Keith-Lucas, Alan 65
Kesey, Ken 42, 133
Kingdom of God 121, 122
knowledge 32f., 87f. *et passim*
Koch 21

ladylikeness 40
Lady-with-the-lamp 39, 40
Lain Entralgo, P. 27, 131
Laing, R.D. 87, 137
Lambourne, Robert A. 26, 99, 131, 138
Last Temptation, The 89
Laws, Plato's 27
laity 1, 6, 81
Leary, Paris 106, 139
Le Bon 136
Liebe 75
Leonard, Peter 63, 65, 135
Leonard, P., Corrigan, P. and 57, 59, 60, 135
liberation 59, 121f.
liberation theology 13, 120–3
life 26, 30, 51, 70, 72, 77, 78, 102, 110
limitation 48, 50, 89f.
Lincoln, Abraham 55, 134
Lodge, David 128
Longfellow, Henry 39, 45
love 7–13, 71, 123f. *et passim*

Machiavellian 61, 64
Mack, J.A. 129
Maimonides 74

Index

male 36–8, 79, 108; disciples 110; nurses 38, 79; societies 110; superiority 37, 38
Man for Himself 71
manipulation 6, 49, 56, 66, 68, 80, 113
Marx, Karl 20
Marxism 59, 68, 119, 122, 123
Marxist social work 10, 60
Maslow, A.H. 138
Mathers, J. and Melinsky, M.A.H. 138
May, William F. 92, 102, 103, 105, 139
Mayer, J.E. and Timms, Noel 52, 130, 134
medical dominance 18f.; ethics 20, 102
medical relationship, the 29, 111
Melinsky, M.A.H. 131
Melinsky, M.A.H., Mathers, J. and 138
McDermott, F. 136
McFarlane, E.A. 133
McGlew, T. and Robertson, A. 130
McKeown, Thomas 17, 20, 130
MacKintosh, J., Dingwall, R. and 132, 133
MacNeice, Louis 87, 138
mediation 84, 111, 114, 126; model 63
Minahan, A., Pincus, A. and 54, 55, 134
minimalism 55f, 104
'miracle drugs' 21
Mirage of Health 21
Miranda, J.P. 140
Miteinanderfühlen 75
Mitgefühl 75
moderated love 125f. *et passim*
moderators 84f.
Moltmann, Jürgen 90
Moltmann-Wendel, Elizabeth 109, 139
morality 120f. *et passim*
mortality 28, 109, 111
mother 34, 35, 39, 42, 86, 110, 112; inadequate 91
mother–child relationship 41
motivation 7f, 71, 75, 79, 88, 105, 114, 117, 119
Muff, Janet 132
Muir Edwin 85, 86, 111, 112, 115, 119, 127, 137, 140, 141
mutuality 32, 35, 49, 50, 61, 75, 81, 82, 90, 92f, 102, 111, 120

Nachgefühl 75
National Association of Social Workers (USA) code of ethics 70

National Asylum Workers Union Magazine 46
national psychology 58
national social policy 55
nationalism 121, 127
Nature and Destiny of Man, The 120
Nature of Sympathy, The 71, 75
Niebuhr, Reinhold 119, 120, 121, 122, 123, 127, 137, 140
Nightingale, Florence 40, 70, 78, 80
Nightingale Pledge 78
Nightingale reforms 36, 39
'noble savage' 97
Norwich, Dame Julian of 89
nurse, nursing 34ff. *et passim*
Nurses Registration Act 36
nurse–patient relationship 41–51, 112
Nuttall, P. 132
Nygren, Anders 73, 136

Oath of Hippocrates 79
occupation 5, 19, 36, 37, 83, 84
obedience 103, 124
objectives 56, 62
obligation 72, 75, 103, 104, 117, 118
Oleson, V., Whittaker, E. and 39, 132
Oliver, J.H. 131
omnipotence 91
omniscience 90, 91
One Flew Over the Cuckoo's Nest 42
'One Foot in Eden' 115, 127
oppressed, the 85, 91, 121f.
Orem, Dorothea E. 43, 44, 46, 133
Orwell, George 80
Osler, Sir William 34
Outka, G. 136
over-commitment 105, 106

parables 108, 119
paradigm of love 9, 125
Parry, N. and Parry, J. 130
Parsons, Talcott 19
particularity 90f.
partly compensatory system 43
passion 120, 121; Christ's 89
Pasteur, Louis 21
Patient as Person 102
Pearson, Geoffrey 61, 63, 130, 135
Pellegrino, E.D. 17
Pellegrino, E.D. and Thomasma, D.S. 28, 130, 131
People not Cases 56
Personal and the Political, The 7, 9

Index

Personal Service Society, The 7, 9, 12, 125
personalist 64
philanthropia 27
philia 28, 32, 73, 74, 81f, 114
Philosophical Basis of Medical Practice, A 28
philosophy 116; Greek 27; social 117
philotechnia 27
Pincus, A. and Minahan, A. 54, 55, 134
Plato's *Laws* 27
Pledge for Nurses 70
political theology 121
politics 9f., 34f.
politics of love 13, 113, **115f.**
Politics of Social Services, The 58
Poor Law 41, 94, 113
power, medical 17f.
pragmatism 123
prayer 99
'Prayer before birth' 87
Prayer of a Physician 74
Precepts, Hippocratic 27
presence 92, 99, 111, 112
priest 8, 25, 106
professional care as love 7
professionalism 3
Professional Power and Social Welfare 6
Professions and Power 19
Prophet, The 78
prophetic role of medicine 84
psyche 96, 105
psychoanalytic approach 71, 72, 110, 113
psychotherapy 8, 52, 92
psychiatry 27, 29, 30, 94
psychology 6, 8, 58, 65, 74
psychosomatic influence 96

quality of life 22
quality of relationship 79
quasi-sexual desire 80

racism 35, 79
radicals 60–4
Radicals in Social Work 57
radical critique of social work 56f., 61–3
Radical Social Service Workers, code of ethics 60
radical social work 56, 60, 126
Ragg, Nicholas 56, 65, 66, 134, 135
Ramsey, Paul 102, 104, 139
reciprocity 102, 105f., 117

reconciliation 30, 98, 125
reform 60–2, 119
reforms, Nightingale 36, 39
reformers, social 13
Register of Nurses, General 79
registration of nurses 36
religious attitude or belief 14, 78, 85, 99, 121, 123
resources 50, 55; maldistribution of 32, 119
respect 6, 42, 70, 72, 80, 109
'restoring the stranger' 29f.
resurrection 85, 94, 98
revelation 14, 74, 90, 92
revolution 59, 60–4, 68, 90, 122
Reynolds, Bertha 52, 134
Rhodes, Philip 22, 131
rights 103, 113, 117, 119
risks 48, 50, 82, 126, 127
ritual 100; of clinic 99
Robertson, A., McGlew, T. and 130
Rogers, Carl 92
Role of Medicine: Dream, Mirage or Nemesis, The 20
Rousseau, J. 75
Russell, A. 128

sacrament 25, 99, 101, 111–14, 126
salvation 105, 116, 117, 122
Santa Filomena 39
saviour, doctor as 22, 23
Scheler, Max 71, 74, 75, 76, 77, 78, 79, 81, 82, 92, 98, 136, 138
science as prophecy 30f.
secular religion 100
self-love 12f., 71f.
sensuality 108, 109
sensuousness 108, 109
Serapion, Hymn of 22, 79
sexism 34f.
Sexton, A. 26, 131
sexuality 110f.
Shaw, George Bernard 6, 23, 70, 129, 131
'Shield of Achilles, The' 68, 115, 123
Sheridan Smith, A.M. 131
Siirala, Aarne 26, 30, 131, 132
sin 72–4, 95, 115, 116, 119, 120, 122
social work 52f. *et passim*
Social Work Practice: Model and Method 54
Social Work Practice under Capitalism: A Marxist Approach 57

Index

Social Work with Undervalued Groups
    15, 56
somatopsychic influence   96
Soyer, David   136
spontaneity   106–8
Statham, Daphne   57, 59, 135
Steinbeck, John   139
Stevens, Barbara   44, 48, 133, 135
stigmatization   112, 118
Stockwell, Barbara   47, 48, 133, 134
Sutherland, M.B.   132
Suttie, Ian D.   34, 110, 132, 139
symbiosis   72
symbols   85, 126, 127; archetypal   105;
    Christian   86, 90
Synoptic passion narrative   89
systems   55, 113

'taboo on tenderness'   110
'Taboo' on Tenderness, The   34
Tagore, Rabindranath   78, 137
'target system'   55
task   47, 48, 54, 105, 126
technique   8, 11, 51, 82
technology   31, 56, 98
Telfer, E., Downie, R.S. and   136
Temkin, O. and Temkin, C.L.   131, 137
tenderness   6, 34, 42, 111
theologians   13, 26, 72, 73, 102, 119,
    122, 123
theology of love   10f.
therapy   1, 8, 26, 45, 61, 66, 111, 126
Thomasma, D.S.   17
Thomasma, D.S., Pellegrino, E.D. and
    28, 130, 131
Tillich, Paul   71, 73f, 79, 82, 98, 136
Timms, Noel, Mayer, J.E. and   52, 130,
    134
Timms, Noel and Watson, D.   135
Titmuss, Richard   6, 116, 117, 118, 123,
    129, 140
Tolstoy, Leo   23, 131
touching   29, 101, 110
Townsend, P. and Davidson, N.   141
training   7, 18, 37, 40, 79, 82, 94
transcendence   3, 11, 14, 26, 51, 74, 77,
    86, 99, 101, 111, 112, 114, 118, 125, 126
Transfiguration', 'The   127
transformation   12, 64, 99, 116

trauma of illness   41
triumphalism, Christian   123
trust   14, 19, 111

'ultra-obligations'   118
UN Declaration of Human Rights   118
unilateral transfer   117
uniqueness   61, 82, 83
unpopular patient   45, 48, 50, 112
Unpopular Patient, The   47
value   73f., 81f., 111f.
Value of Medicine, The   22
Vanier, Jean   48, 134
verbalization   37, 112
Veruysen, Margaret Connor   133
vicarious feeling   75, 76, 81, 82
victims   61, 67, 90
Vidales, R.   122
Vidales, R. and Gibellini, R.   140
vision   29, 76, 98, 111, 114
vocation   2, 11, 15, 70, 77, 107
Voice of Illness, The   26
voluntary agencies   53, 55, 59
vulnerability   1, 2, 14, 28, 32, 41, 52,
    84, 88, 90, 93, 108, 124, 126

Watson, David   117, 118, 123, 130, 140
Watson, David, Timms, Noel and   135
weakness   57, 84, 109, 111
wealth   7, 32, 57, 63, 119
welfare   1, 5, 52, 64, 70, 81, 88, 89, 104,
    113, 114, 116, 117, 118
well-being   28, 31, 32, 54, 58, 59, 92,
    96, 98
White, R.   40, 133
Whittaker, E. and Oleson, V.   39, 132
'wholly compensatory system'   43
Wilding, Paul   6, 7, 128, 129, 130, 135
Wilkes, Ruth   15, 16, 56, 60, 65, 66, 83,
    130, 134, 135, 136, 137
Williams, Daniel Day   98, 101, 115, 119,
    138, 139, 140
Williams, Katherine   44, 133
Wilson, Michael   20, 21, 98, 130, 131
Wolters, C.   138
women   23, 31, 34, 36–42, 50, 79, 108–10
working class   59–62
worship   99

Yeats, W.B.   64, 135